MANUAL

safe
sex

MANUAL OF safe sex

DONALD KILBY, M.D.

Student Health Services
University of Ottawa
Ottawa, Ontario

B.C. Decker Inc • Toronto • Philadelphia

Publisher

B.C. Decker Inc.
3228 South Service Road
Burlington, Ontario   L7N 3H8

B.C. Decker Inc.
P.O. Box 30246
Philadelphia, Pennsylvania   19103

Sales and Distribution

United States and Possessions	**The C.V. Mosby Company** 11830 Westline Industrial Drive Saint Louis, Missouri 63146
Canada	**The C.V. Mosby Company, Ltd.** 5240 Finch Avenue East, Unit No. 1 Scarborough, Ontario M1S 4P2
United Kingdom, Europe and the Middle East	**Blackwell Scientific Publications, Ltd.** Osney Mead, Oxford OX2 OEL, England
Australia	**Holt-Saunders Pty. Limited** 9 Waltham Street Artarmon, N.S.W. 2064 Australia
Japan	**Igaku-Shoin Ltd.** Tokyo International P.O. Box 5063 1-28-36 Hongo, Bunkyo-ku, Tokyo 113, Japan
Asia	**Holt-Saunders Asia Limited** 10/F, Inter-Continental Plaza Tsim Sha Tsui East Kowloon, Hong Kong

Manual of Safe Sex   ISBN 1-55009-016-X

Library of Congress catalog card number: 86-71435

Printed in Singapore   10 9 8 7 6 5 4 3 2 1

INTRODUCTION

As a society we have evolved. We have greater respect for others, regardless of race, sex or creed. We have become more tolerant and more eager to protect their human rights as well as our own.

Changes in social behavior and social tolerance have also altered the way we feel about ourselves and our sexuality. Sexual expression has changed since we have been trying to drop that old double standard and since women have discovered sexual freedom. Oral contraceptives have allowed them to avoid unwanted pregnancies and to carefully map their goals so as to be fulfilled in this area. As well, the moment for starting a family can be a planned event.

Conversely, the sexual revolution has seen more and more people having more and more casual encounters. There have been more teenage pregnancies, more abortions, and more sexually transmitted diseases. This is not the place to debate the moral issues of sexual promiscuity, abortion, teenage sex, or open relationships. These are best left to others.

However as a physician, I feel we should examine the impact of this sexual revolution on our health. The number of unwanted pregnancies and the increasing prevalence of sexually transmitted diseases among all social groups is proof enough that sexually active teenagers as well as many adults are ill prepared to undertake responsible, sexually active lives. This is through no fault of their own, in most cases. I hope readers will appreciate the need for organized instruction through the educational system, so that in the future, teenagers and young adults will be better informed.

In this text I will develop the theme of "Safe Sex". As we emerge from the era of sexual freedom and sexual revolution, we must stop to look at the impact of changing sexual behavior. The reader will be impressed by the growing proportion of illness associated with increased number of casual sexual relationships. The reader will also see that even though contraception is important in avoiding unwanted pregnancies and allowing for sexual encounters for pleasure, protecting oneself and one's partner from the ever-growing threat of sexually transmitted disease is equally important.

The rules of safe sex are few; their application will allow for intimacy and will help the sexually active to avoid unwanted pregnancies, thereby reducing the number of abortions in our society. These rules will also reduce the risk of acquiring a sexually transmitted disease, be it as common as gonorrhea or as threatening as AIDS.

The information in this teaching guide is relevant to the young, who will benefit the most; to their parents, so that they too, can counsel their children; and to educators everywhere, whose job it is to properly inform the uninformed. Any words or acronyms requiring definition or explanation may be found in the glossary.

Any meaningful discussion of contraception or sexually transmitted diseases should take place after basic knowledge of human sexual anatomy and physiology has been acquired. To this end, the following section will look at the internal and external anatomy of both the male and female genitalia as well as the functioning of each.

After reading this book, the reader will find that safe sex means different things for different people. For committed heterosexual couples, it may be that safe sex means the effective use of a contraceptive method. For the uncommitted heterosexual, it should mean effective contraception and sexual practices that limit the acquisition or spread of STDs.

Homosexuals in particular, because of their sexual practices and their high risk of acquiring AIDS through such practices, should engage in unprotected sexual intimacy only after they have proven to themselves that they are infection free. Heterosexuals and homosexuals alike should limit the number of sexual contacts.

In conclusion, if you intend to have casual sexual encounters, or if you have only recently met your sexual partner, you should practice safe sex. The term has significance beyond the consideration of contraception. The following steps will help safeguard you and your partners.

1. Do not exhange body fluids—do not take sperm orally, vaginally or rectally. Ejaculate should be passed only into a condom.

2. Avoid oral-genital contacts.
3. Avoid oral-anal contacts.
4. Avoid genital-anal contacts.
5. Wash thoroughly before engaging in sexual intimacy.
6. Use a mechanical barrier such as a condom.
7. Even if your partner says he or she is safe, insist that safe sex be practiced.
8. Wash after sexual intercourse.
9. If any casual or new sexual partner is unwilling to follow the above conditions, LEARN TO SAY NO!

It is this author's recommendation that these sexual practices should not be encouraged. They should be kept only for those people who are truly committed to each other. Only between healthy infection-free individuals does more exotic sexual behavior carry a margin of safety.

CONTENTS

MALE GENITALIA

The male reproductive organs have multiple purposes. They excrete urine, are responsible for reproduction by way of the production and distribution of sperm and are erogenous areas, sites of sexual pleasure. They may also become reservoirs for sexually transmitted disease.

External Genitalia

Male external sex organs include the penis and the scrotum. The testicles and their attachments, even though they are contained in the scrotum, are usually considered internal organs.

Penis

The penis, from the Latin word for ''tail'', is a cylindrical structure containing the urethra and a system of erectile tissue. There are three elongated bodies that course the length of the penis. The two corpora cavernosa run parallel along the top of the penis, while the corpus spongiosum runs along the underside through its full length. The urethra is housed within the corpus spongiosum. The urethra is a duct that originates in the bladder and releases urine and semen. These three erectile compartments, or spongy bodies, fill with blood during sexual excitement, causing the penis to become erect. A system of valves prevents blood flow from leaving the penis until the stimulus subsides. Then the blood quickly leaves the penis, permitting it to return to its flaccid state.

The skin covering the penis is loose, allowing for the increased length of the penis during erection. The skin normally covering the glans, or head, of the flaccid penis is called the foreskin or prepuce. During erection it is pulled back to expose the head of the penis. The glans, Latin for ''acorn'', is an extension of the corpus spongiosum and contains the urethra's external opening. It is the most sensitive area of the penis. The underside of the glans is attached to the foreskin by a thin band of tissue called the frenulum.

Glands round the rim of the glans secrete smegma, which often becomes trapped between the glans and the foreskin. This smegma is responsible for a cheeselike secretion with a distinct odor, which can easily be controlled by careful washing.

A circumcision is an operation to remove the foreskin (Fig 1-1).This may be necessary because the foreskin is too tight around the glans, or because of repeated infections, or for religious or personal reasons. For circumcised men, the glans of the penis is always exposed. There is no difference in the sexual abilities of circumcised and uncircumcised men. Nor does penile size have anything whatsoever to do with sexual function. The average flaccid penis measures three to four inches, while the average erect penis measures five to seven inches. Preoccupation with penile size is unwarranted, nor is the organ's size a gauge of fertility.

Scrotum

The scrotum serves as a pouch for the testicles. It is located at the base of the penis between the thighs. The skin is usually darker than the body skin and contains many sweat glands. It normally hangs loosely if warm and relaxed. But if exposed to cold, and sometimes during sexual stimulation, small muscles within the walls of the scrotum cause the skin to wrinkle, pushing the testicles upward towards the abdominal cavity for warmth, or out of the way during sexual play. Inside, the scrotum is divided into two compartments, each containing one testicle and its spermatic cord.

When palpating the scrotum, one can feel at the superior pole of the testicle ''cordlike'' structures that make up the spermatic cord. They are the vasa deferentia, tubes that carry sperm; blood vessels, a vein and an artery; and a nerve and a muscle. The cremasteric muscles are used to pull the testicles up closer to the abdomen in response to certain stimuli, as mentioned earlier.

For the most part the scrotum acts as a sort of thermostat. During fetal development, the testicles move down from the

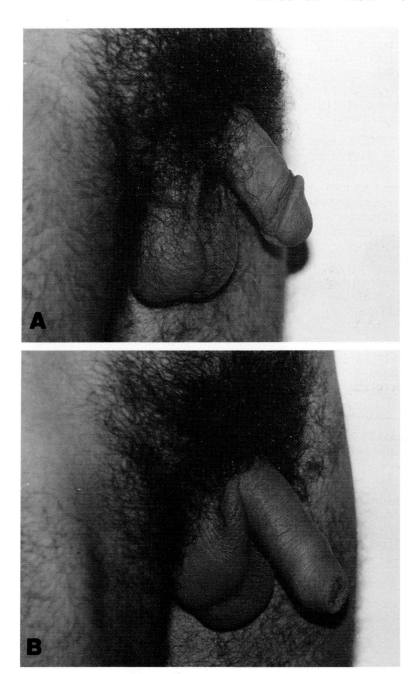

Figure 1–1 Male external genitalia. *A*, Circumcised and *B*, uncircumcised penis.

abdominal cavity, through the inguinal canals to hang inside the scrotum. If they were to remain in the abdomen, the body's relatively high temperature would not favor the production of sperm. Since the testicles are in the scrotum and are free to move closer or farther away from the body core, an even temperature is provided for continuous production of healthy sperm. This function is accomplished by the cremasteric and scrotal muscles.

Internal Genitalia

Testicles

The testicles have two major functions: the production of both the male hormone, testosterone, and of spermatozoa. There are normally two testicles, one in each side of the scrotum. Absence of one testicle may be a congenital variance or may indicate a failure of that testicle to descend from the abdominal cavity into the scrotum during fetal development. This can be surgically corrected in childhood. The testicles are smooth, oval-shaped and measure about one and a half inches in length. The left testicle usually hangs a little lower than the right. See figure 1-2 for the male reproductive organs and Figure 1-3 for a sagittal section of a testis.

Sperm Production

Within the testicle are numerous lobes, in which are located many tubules. Sperm is produced within these tubules via a process called spermatogenesis (Fig. 1-4). The sperm gather at the back side of the testicle in a collecting system called the vasa efferentia. Sperm production begins at puberty and continues throughout a man's life. It takes 64 days for the complete production of sperm, which goes on continuously in three stages.

Stage 1

Cells called spermatogonia, at the outer border of these seminiferous tubules, enlarge to form ''primary spermatocytes,'' or cells.

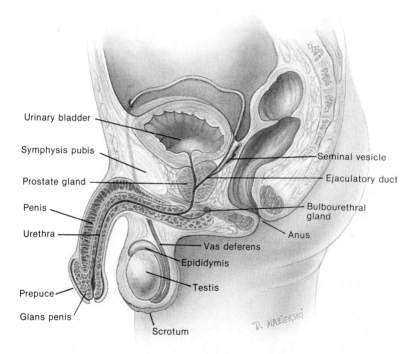

Figure 1-2 External and internal male genitalia: section through pelvis, seen from side.

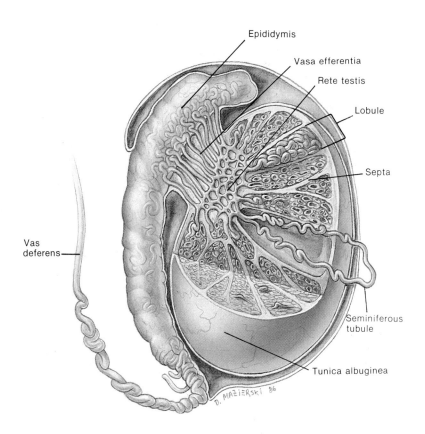

Figure 1-3 Sagittal section of a testis.

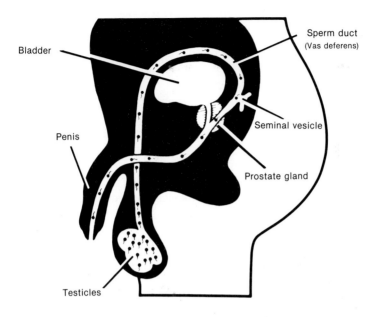

Figure 1–4 Male reproductive organs. (Reproduced with permission of Wyeth Ltd.)

Stage 2

Chromosomes in each primary spermatocyte replicate; then the cell divides into two "secondary spermatocytes," each containing 46 chromosomes.

Stage 3

The secondary spermatocytes undergo meiotic division, i.e. without chromosomal division, resulting in two spermatids, each with 23 chromosomes. One spermatid contains the X chromosome, the other contains the Y chromosome for sexual differentiation.

Therefore sperm contains an X chromosome or a Y chromosome and 22 other chromosomes. The X-chromosome-bearing sperm will help to produce females at fertilization with the female ovum, while the Y will help to produce males.

Each spermatid elongates to become spermatozoon, which later mature to spermatozoa. These mature sperm are passed from the testicle to the epididymis. At this stage, they are still non-motile. They will remain in the epididymis for between 18 hours and 10 days. There they will develop motility and become capable of fertilizing the ovum.

Epididymides

The epididymides are collecting tubes located at the superior pole of the testicles. Each epididymis, one for each testicle, is about 20 feet long. It is a twisted convoluted mass not to be confused with the artery or vein also located in this area.

Vasa Deferentia

A small quantity of sperm is stored in the epididymis of each testicle, but probably most is stored in the vas deferens of each. They can remain stored, maintaining their fertility, for up to 42 days, though with normal sexual activity, such prolonged storage probably does not occur. During vasectomy, the vasa deferentia are transsected and ligated, cutting off further supply of mature spermatozoa to the ejaculatory ducts, rendering the man sterile.

The ampullae of the vasa deferentia join the ducts of two other saclike organs called the seminal vesicles. Together they form the ejaculatory ducts that run inside the prostate gland to join the urethra. Prior to ejaculation, movement of sperm is passive. Once they mix with other secretions to make up the semen, the sperm use their long tails to swim vigorously.

Urethra

The urethra is a long tubelike structure that courses from the bladder through the prostate, ending at the tip of the glans. It serves to transport urine and semen. Because of an intricate valve system formed by certain muscles, semen and urine cannot be released together to the outside. Semen enters the urethra through the ejaculatory ducts described above.

Seminal Vesicles

These are two saclike structures located near the ampullae of the vasa deferentia, just superior to the prostate and posterior to the bladder. These provide seminal fluid, along with the prostate, which helps give spermatozoa the motility necessary for fertilization of the ovum. The seminal vesicles ensure a large volume of semen as well as adding fructose and other substances that have both nutrient and protective value for the ejaculated sperm.

Prostate Gland

This is a small firm structure the size of a chestnut, through which the male urethra, as well as the two ejaculatory ducts, must course. During ejaculation a thin milky fluid is secreted from the prostate to combine with the semen. It is alkaline (basic), and by altering the pH of the vagina, it probably helps to ensure normal sperm motility and fertility.

Bulbourethral Glands (Cowper's Glands)

These two pea-sized glands, also known as Cowper's glands, are located just below the prostate. During sexual excitement they secrete a clear alkaline fluid into the urethra. This is usually felt at the tip of the penis as a clear, viscous substance. The fluid may contain some sperm cells and, therefore, may account for the high rate of pregnancy when coitus interruptus is used as contraception, i.e., withdrawal of the penis from the vagina prior to ejaculation.

In summary, the ejaculated semen contains sperm cells combined with secretions from the seminal vesicles, the prostate and the bulbourethral glands. It usually has a volume of a little less than a teaspoon and is not harmful to the vagina or if ingested, except in the presence of a sexually transmitted disease. It is greyish white in color, the consistency varying according to the frequency of ejaculation. Each cubic centimeter or milliliter of semen contains an average 120 million sperm. This means that in an average three to four cubic centimeters of sperm per ejaculation, there are 400 to 500 million sperm. A man is considered infertile if there are less than 35,000,000 sperm per milliliter, or if greater than 25 percent of the sperm are abnormally shaped, having two heads, two tails or impaired motility.

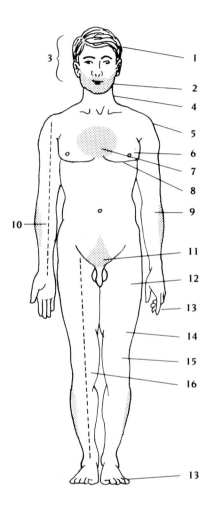

Figure 1-5 The secondary sexual characteristics of the male. On the average, taller and heavier than the female. **1.** *Head hair*: may fall out with age. **2.** *Facial hair*: grows throughout adult life. **3.** *Features*: more pronounced, face longer, head (front to back) longer. **4.** *Neck*: thicker, longer, larynx one-third larger. **5.** *Shoulders*: broader, squarer. **6.** *Chest*: larger in every dimension. **7.** *Body hair*: more evident, especially on chest and arms. **8.** *Breasts*: rudimentary in size. **9.** *Muscles*: bigger, more obvious. **10.** *Arms*: longer, thicker, ''carrying angle'' straight. **11.** *Pubic hair*: growing up to a point, forming triangle. **12.** *Hips*: narrower. **13.** *Hands and feet*: larger, fingers and toes stronger and blunter. **14.** *Thighs*: more cylindrical with bulge of muscles. **15.** *Legs*: longer, bulging calves. **16.** *Angle of thigh and leg*: as with ''carrying angle'' of arm, forming straight line, thigh to ankle. (Adapted with permission from Haeberrle IJ. The sex atlas New York: Seabury Press. p. 20)

Male Hormone Production by the Testes

Male hormones are called androgens. These are produced in the testes by the interstitial Leydig cells, these cells developing until puberty, by which time they are more numerous. The main male hormone is testosterone, which is responsible for the development of secondary sexual characteristics (Fig. 1-5). Male hormones are needed for a man to develop full sexual potential. However, in adult males their presence is not required for normal sexual function.

The pituitary gland in the brain secretes the gonadotrophic hormones LH, luteinizing hormone, and FSH, follicle stimulating hormone. These play a major role in controlling male sexual functions. LH is primarily responsible for testosterone production; FSH, for spermatogenesis, or production of sperm. Both are needed, however, for spermatogenesis to occur, and FSH greatly potentiates LH in promoting testosterone production. LH and FSH secretions from the pituitary gland are dictated by the hypothalamus, a small gland located in the brain near the pituitary. By a mechanism of feedback control, high levels of testosterone act on the hypothalamus, which then has an inhibitory effect on the pituitary, causing a reduction of LH and FSH; therefore, the testes gradually decrease testosterone production. The mechanism also works in the opposite way to protect against too little production of testosterone. Thus an optimal level of circulating hormone is always maintained. Until puberty, the hypothalamus inhibits production of testosterone. Then, for reasons as yet poorly understood, at puberty the gland loses its inhibitory sensivity, allowing for increased testosterone production and spermatogenesis.

Men are able to secrete testosterone and produce sperm until death. However, most do experience slowly decreasing function in their 40s or 50s. A small group of men may even experience symptoms of menopause similar to those of women.

FEMALE GENITALIA

2

Like the male reproductive organs, the female sex organs serve other functions, including that of realizing orgasmic potential.

External Female Genitalia

Collectively this area is known as the vulva, Latin for "covering." See Figure 2-1.

Mons Pubis

The mons pubis, or mons veneris, Latin for "mountain of venus," consists of fatty tissue overlying the pubic bone. The area is covered with pubic hair, becoming the most prominent part of the vulva.

Labia Majora

The labia majora, or "larger lips", when not stimulated sexually, close in the midline to protect underlying structures: the labia minora, urethra, clitoris and vaginal opening. They are thick fatty folds of skin that extend from the mons pubis anteriorly downward.

Labia Minora

Just inside the labia majora are two smaller and thinner fatty folds of skin called the labia minora. They come to the midline to drape over the vaginal opening, urethra and clitoris. At the anterior, or top portion, the labia minora merge to form a hood over the clitoris.

Clitoris

Just below the mons pubis, at that point where the labia minora merge, is the clitoris, from the Greek Kleitoris, or "that which is closed in." It is a short cylindrical organ composed erectile tissue much like the penis. This spongy tissue becomes engorged during sexual stimulation, causing the clitoris to increase in size. The organ is unique, totally committed in its physiological function to initiating or elevating sexual tension. There are no male counterparts. It is very sensitive to the touch.

The clitoris is covered by a hood or preskin. Because of the close relationship of the tissues, smegma may accumulate in the area, causing irritation and, occasionally, other difficulties.

Bartholin Glands

The Bartholin glands are situated in each of the minor labia. Their ducts are located on the inner surfaces of the labia, adjacent to the vaginal opening. Late in the excitement phase of sexual tension, these glands secrete a mucoid material for introital lubrication. They do not, however, provide sufficient secretion for vaginal lubrication. They may become infected, thus causing pain and swelling.

Urethra

Just below the clitoris, but above the vaginal introitus, is the urethral opening, which carries urine from the bladder to the outside. In women its course is very short. Because of where it is situated and because of its length, it is quite vulnerable, allowing any organisms in the area to make their way up its length to the bladder. This explains why women have more urinary tract infections of both the urethra and bladder than men. Stimulation by the penis during first sexual encounters may explain the phenomenon of "honeymoon cystitis," a condition marked by more frequent urination, pain on urination and bladder discomfort.

Vaginal Opening

Below the urethra is the vaginal opening. Prior to first intercourse it may be partially closed by a thin membrane known as the hymen. However, usually by first intercourse the hymen is but a ring of tissue; its central opening is needed to release menstrual flow. Therefore, it is a fallacy that a virgin has an un-perforated hymen. If the hymen remained intact at puberty, menstrual flow would accumulate behind it. However, the hymenal ring may tear during intercourse, causing bleeding and some discomfort.

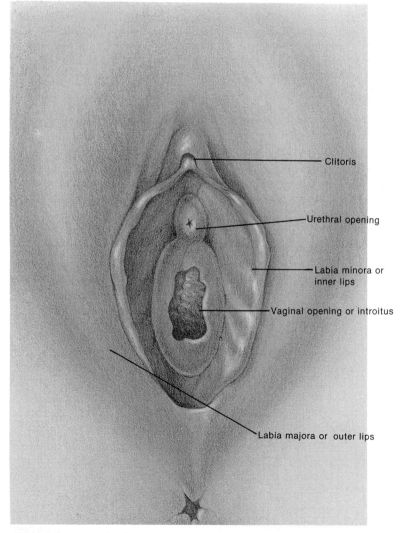

Figure 2–1 Female external sexual organs.

Internal Female Genitalia

Vagina

The vagina, Latin for "sheath", is a long cylinder measuring about three to four inches. (See Figure 2-2 for a diagrammatic representation of the female internal reproductive organs.) It extends from the vaginal opening to the cervix and it serves multiple purposes, namely:

1. Providing the primary physical means of manifesting female heterosexuality. The vagina also serves as a receptacle for the man's penis and ejaculated semen which then moves on to the uterus through the cervix for conception.
2. Serving as a birth canal from the uterus to outside.
3. Providing a passageway for menstrual flow from the uterus to the outside.

The vaginal walls are moist and are normally in contact, except where the cervix protrudes into its cavity. The walls are thick and arranged in a number of transverse folds known as vaginal rugae. Usually, physiological vaginal secretions do not escape to the outside. Some women may have a vaginal discharge consisting of normal secretions. If this discharge is unusual in color, odor or consistency, it may represent disease and is often the first sign of infection, be it sexually acquired or otherwise.

The vagina itself has no glands; its surface is moistened by the cervical glands and to some extent by transudation from its own surface. These secretions are usually acidic, a property derived from organisms or from normal vaginal flora that produce lactic acid. Changes in normal vaginal flora are the result of infection from competitive organisms. These organisms will be further discussed in the chapter "Vaginitis." Since different organisms live in a healthy balance within the vagina, sprays and douches should be avoided. Tampons should also be changed frequently.

During sexual stimulation, the vaginal vault becomes lubricated to allow for easy penetration of the penis. It can also adjust to accommodate any penis size. Only the vaginal opening seems unaccommodating, as it may be too "tight" if the muscle in the area is not relaxed or the hymenal ring not yet torn. It may also seem "too loose" for some women after childbirth or as a normal process of aging. Vaginal muscles may be controlled to allow for adequate relaxation and appropriate contraction during intercourse. Exercise programs that increase muscle tone in this area are helpful.

Cervix

The cervix protrudes into the vagina at its deepest end. It is really part of the uterus. Its central canal, or cervical mouth, opens into the inner uterus and provides a passageway for

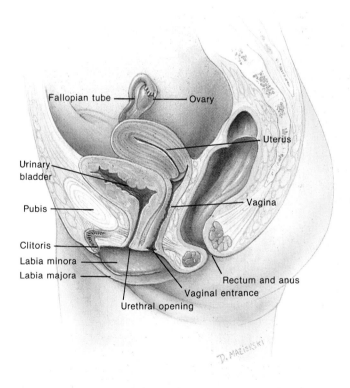

Figure 2–2   Female internal reproductive organs.

sperm to enter the uterus and for menstrual flow to leave the uterus at the end of each hormonal cycle. Cancer of the cervix may be detected early by routine examination and Papanicolaou (PAP) tests.

Uterus

The uterus, Latin for "womb", is a single muscular organ the size of a small pear, located in the midline of the pelvis between the bladder at the front and the rectum behind. On either side of the uterus are the fallopian tubes and the ovaries. In women who have never had children, the organ is approximately three inches long. It has the ability to increase dramatically in size during pregnancy and undergoes involution or reduction in size after menopause.

For descriptive purposes, the uterus is divided into the following parts: the fundus, the body, the isthmus and the cervix.

The fallopian tubes open into the uterine cavity at the up per end of each lateral margin. The cavity is small, owing to the thickness of the uterine walls. The inner lining is known as the endometrium, which responds to various changes in hormonal concentrations during the menstrual cycle. If fertilization does not occur or if oral contraceptives are discontinued, the endometrium's superficial layer is sloughed off and discharged at menstruation. Ruptured vessels produce the bleeding that is the menstrual flow. A deeper layer remains to establish new endometrium in the next cycle. If fertilization occurs, the dividing cells that make up the fetus become embedded in the endometrium to establish a pregnancy.

The uterus is usually tilted forward over the urinary bladder. Occasionally, however, it may tilt backwards, i.e., retroverted. This can make examination more difficult and may cause clinical complaints.

Fallopian Tubes

The fallopian tubes, named after the sixteenth century Italian anatomist, Fallopius, are more adequately described as oviducts, which means "paths of the eggs". Each tube provides a passageway for the egg after it leaves the ovary on its way to the uterus. Sperm can also use this passageway to meet the egg en route for fertilization. If the tubes have been damaged by previous infection, the fertilized egg may implant in the fallopian tube. This is known as an ectopic pregnancy, and it must be terminated surgically.

Each fallopian tube is about four inches, or 10 centimeters, in length and opens into the uterine cavity. The abdominal orifice remains free, opening into the abdominal cavity close to the ovary. The tube's wide ovarian end has fingerlike extensions called fimbriae that move across the surface of the ovary. Their function is to catch the ovum after it is released from the ovary's surface and to sweep it into the tube. If the egg is not caught, it becomes lost in the peritoneal cavity; that is, within the abdomen.

At least one of the uterine tubes must be patent, or accessible, for pregnancy to occur. If neither tube is patent, sterility occurs. The most common cause of blockage is inflammation as a result of sexually transmitted infection.

Ovaries

The ovaries, or female gonads, are almond-sized organs on either side of the uterus. Much like the testicles, the ovaries serve two functions: they produce ova, eggs, as well as the hormones estrogen and progesterone, which are secreted directly into the bloodstream.

Production of Ova

At birth approximately 500,000 primordial follicles, or immature ova, are present. However, only about 375 of these go on to develop sufficiently to be expelled at cyclical ovulations. These monthly ovulations are brought about by rhythmic changes in the rates of secretion of sex hormones and corresponding changes in the sex organs themselves. This is known as the female sexual cycle. The average duration of a cycle is 28 days, but it may range from 20 to 45 days.

The 500,000 primordial follicles are known as oocytes (Fig. 2-3). They remain in a state of suspended development until puberty. At that time one or more oocytes develop into mature ova, or eggs, each month. An ova will be produced by one or the other ovary. There does not seem to be any set pattern as to which ovary will produce an egg during any given cycle. This procedure will continue until menopause.

Under hormonal influence, an oocyte that lies beneath the outer layer of the ovary, within a cluster of cells, grows to a point where it appears as a sort of vesicle or blister called a graafian follicle. This follicle undergoes further development so that the primary oocyte, which contains 46 chromosomes, including two X chromosomes) divides into two cells, or larger secondary oocytes, as well as into a small "polar body" containing 23 chromosomes. Only a secondary oocyte is destined for further maturation. At ovulation the follicle bursts, and this secondary oocyte is expelled into the abdominal cavity, where it is usually picked up by the nearest fallopian tube. Again it divides to reproduce the same number of chromosomes, 23, within a large ootid, or ovum, as well as a second small polar body. After fertilization the polar body is destroyed. The ovum with its 23 chromosomes, including one X, is fertilized by a sperm with its 23 chromosomes, including one X or one Y, to form a new cell or zygote. The zygote now contains 46 chromosomes and a pair of sex chromosomes - XX or XY. A fertilized egg containing XX chromosomes is destined to become a female, whereas one containing XY will become a male.

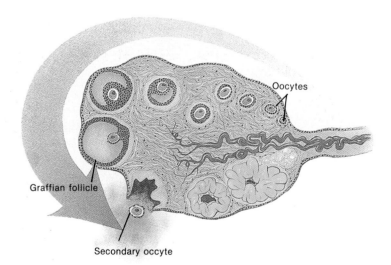

Oocytes

Graffian follicle

Secondary occyte

Figure 2-3   Production of ova. (With permission of Ortho Pharmaceutical Corporation)

The Production of Hormones

The ovaries produce estrogens and progestogens, or female gonadal hormones. Estrogens are responsible for secondary female sexual characteristics, including breast development, typical hair distribution, typical fat distribution, etc. (Fig. 2-4). Progesterone is mostly concerned with the final preparation of the uterus for pregnancy and the breasts for lactation. Sexual hormones are required only for the development of these characteristics and are not needed for normal sexual function. Therefore, women in menopause can expect the same sexual responsiveness as in their reproductive years.

Hormones from the brain control the ovaries' estrogen and progesterone production. Ovulation is not dependant on ovarian hormonal production, but rather is dictated by the production or influence of gonadotropins, the hormones produced by the pituitary gland. They are FSH, follicle stimulating hormone and LH, luteinizing hormone.

There is a continuous interplay between the ovarian hormones estrogen and progesterone, and the pituitary gonadotrophic hormones FSH and LH, causing a rhythmic oscillation of both ovarian and pituitary gonadotrophins. On the one hand, pituitary LH and FSH cause ovarian secretion of estrogen and progesterone. On the other hand, the presence of circulating ovarian hormones inversely affects the pituitary, resulting in a decreased rate of secretion of gonadotrophic hormones, FSH and LH. This is known as a "negative feedback mechanism." Pituitary secretion of FSH and LH is controlled by the hypothalamus, located in proximity to the pituitary gland, or hypophysis, at the base of the brain. Therefore, estrogen and progesterone exert their effect on the hypothalamus, which then works to control secretion of the gonadotrophic hormones by the pituitary gland.

The day prior to ovulation, the pituitary secretes an increased amount of LH, probably because estrogen and progesterone are at low concentrations at this time. Similarly, FSH levels rise during the early part of the month. Estrogen and progesterone increase under the influence of rising FSH and LH, causing the latter to drop off in the second half of the cycle. This decline results in a corresponding decrease in estrogen and progesterone at the end of the cycle, if the egg is not fertilized by the negative feedback mechanism. This drop in ovarian hormones then signals the uterus to shed its superficial lining, causing menstruation. Menstruation occurs around the fourteenth day, after ovulation.

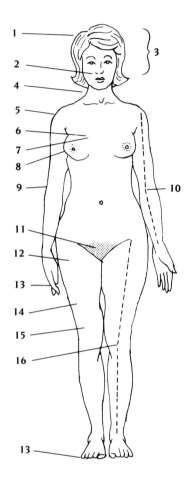

Figure 2-4 The secondary sexual characteristics of the female. On the average, shorter and lighter than the male. **1.** Head hair: more lasting. **2.** Facial hair: very faint, usually noticeable only in later years. **3.** Features: more delicate, face rounder, head smaller, rounder (from top). **4.** Neck: shorter, more rounded, larynx smaller. **5.** Shoulders: more rounded, sloping. **6.** Chest: smaller, narrower. **7.** Body hair: very light and faint. **8.** Breasts: prominent, also well-developed nipples with large surrounding rings. **9.** Muscles: largely hidden under layers of fat. **10.** Arms: "carrying angle" bent. **11.** Pubic hair: forming straight line across at top. **12.** Hips: wider, more rounded. **13.** Hands and feet: smaller and narrower. **14.** Thighs: wider at top and shorter in length. **15.** Legs: shorter with smoother contours. **16.** Angle of thigh and leg: as with "carrying angle" of arm, slightly bent, forming an angle at the knee. (Adapted with permission from Haeberrle IJ. The sex atlas. New York: Seabury Press. p. 20.)

During pregnancy the developing fetus and its placenta produce hormones; the placenta releases a chorionic gonadotrophin shortly after implantation into the uterine wall. This gonadotrophin has a function very similar to that of the luteinizing hormone secreted by the pituitary, causing an increased secretion of estrogen and progesterone. Menstruation does not occur; further ovulations are also halted.

Birth control pills affect the hypothalamic-pituitary-ovarian feedback system in much the same way. As long as estrogens-progesterones are taken via the birth control pill, the brain and the ovaries are made to believe these hormones are derived from a possible pregnancy and, therefore, ovulation does not occur. In order to cause the "artificial menstruation" of the oral contraceptive, the pill is discontinued, bringing about a sudden drop in ovarian hormone levels similar to that occurring prior to natural menstrual flow.

The Menstrual Cycle

The menstrual cycle between puberty and menopause gives a woman her reproductive capacity (Fig. 2-5). It is characterized by the cyclical release of an ovum under gonadotrophic hormone control in preparation for fertilization. It is only in the days surrounding ovulation that a woman can become pregnant. The most constant event by which we can follow this cycle is the menstrual bleeding. It is for this reason that we call it the menstrual cycle.

The first menstrual flow occurs at puberty, usually between 11 and 13 years of age, and is called menarche. Initially menstrual cycles may be irregular and may occur without any warning signals at all. This is attributed to the absence of ovulation with initial cycles or to the sporadic occurrence of ovulations. Adolescents should consider themselves fertile, however, from the onset of first menstrual flow. They cannot rely on "safe" periods throughout their cycle, and especially not on menstruation itself, as spontaneous ovulations in this age group are frequent. In mature women, a definite pattern is established. Cycles are usually 25 to 35 days between menstruation. Some minor irregularity may be normal, but women whose cycles change drastically should seek medical attention to rule out any pathology or disease. As a woman grows older ovarian function decreases. Cycles become more irregular until they stop completely with menopause.

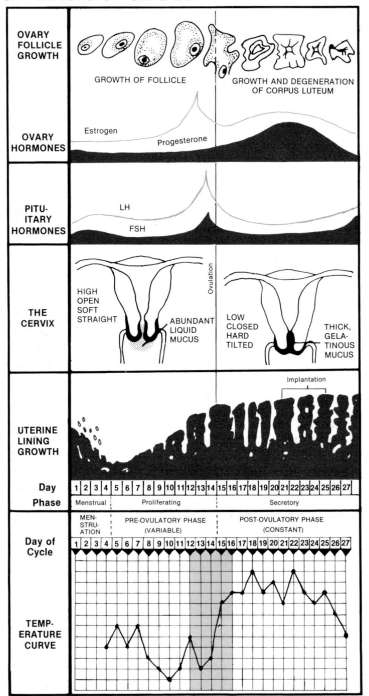

Figure 2–5 The relationships among ovarian activity, ovarian hormones in the bloodstream, the cervix, the mucus, the endometrium and the temperature curve during the menstrual cycle.

The relationship between gonadotrophic hormones, ovarian hormones and ovulation has already been explained. Under the influence of similar cyclical changes in hormones, the lining of the uterus prepares itself each cycle for the possible implantation of a fertilized egg. If no implantation occurs the lining is sloughed off, and the cycle starts over. If implantation does occur, the lining further develops under the influence of feto-placental hormones to sustain the endometrial lining during the entire pregnancy.

Day one of the menstrual cycle is the first day of menstruation, menstrual flow. The last day of the menstrual cycle is the day just preceding the onset of menstruation.

The following discussion starts with the phase following menstruation, approximately day five of the cycle. In this way we can best illustrate the endometrial developments leading to implantation or menstruation.

Proliferative Phase

The proliferative phase, when the endometrium is preparing for ovulation, begins after most of the endometrial lining has been desquamated, sloughed off, by the process of menstruation, at about day five (Fig. 2-6A). Under the influence of estrogen being increasingly secreted into the bloodstream by the ovaries, the endometrial lining starts to proliferate, or thicken.

During this time a graafian follicle is also developing to produce a mature ovum. The ovum is released at approximately day 14 of a 28-day cycle or, more accurately, 14 days prior to menstruation, day 19 of a 33-day cycle. The time between ovulation and menstruation is relatively constant, whereas the time between menstruation and ovulation may vary considerably. At ovulation the lining of the endometrium is thick enough for implantation. Menstruation will only occur if the ovum is not fertilized or is not implanted in the endometrial lining.

Secretory Phase

During the latter half of the menstrual cycle, estrogen and progesterone secretion increase dramatically. At this time hormonal secretion is derived from a mass of cells called corpus luteum, which were left behind on the surface of the ovary after the ovum was released. These hormones cause further thickening of the endometrium (Fig. 2-6B); glands also develop that

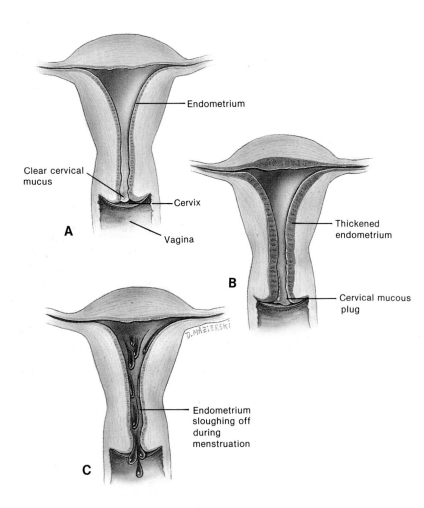

Figure 2–6   The three phases of the menstrual cycle: *A*, proliferative phase, *B*, secretroy phase, and *C*, menstrual phase.

secrete endometrial fluid. Blood vessels increase in size as secretory activity intensifies. The thickness of the lining of the uterus almost doubles during the secretory phase.

The purpose of all these changes is to provide an endometrium containing large amounts of stored nutrients, ensuring an optimal environment for the implanted fertilized ovum of early pregnancy.

During pregnancy the developing fetus and its placenta secrete chorionic gonadotrophic hormones that stimulate the corpus luteum to secrete estrogen and progesterone. As long as the secretion of these hormones is maintained, menstruation and further ovulation cannot occur.

Menstrual Phase

If the ovum is not fertilized, secretion of estrogen and progesterone declines rapidly, approximately two days before the end of the menstrual cycle, causing menstruation to follow. During the hours preceding menstruation, the vessels of the endometrial lining go into spasm, depriving the lining of blood, therefore causing tissue to become necrotic, to die. Hemorrhaging occurs into the outer layer of the endometrium, which then separates from deeper layers, and the menstrual flow starts (Fig. 2-6C). This process of desquamation lasts approximately 48 hours. The desquamated tissue and blood also initiate uterine contractionzs that aid in their expulsion into the vagina. This bloody discharge does not usually clot. If clots are seen at menstruation, they may indicate uterine pathology, or disease. Usually menstrual blood loss is complete after five days.

Further Reading

Anderson JE. Grant's atlas of anatomy. Baltimore: Williams & Wilkins, 1983: Section 3.

Guyton AC. Textbook of medical physiology. Philadelphia: WB Saunders, 1981: 992–1003, 1005–1018, 1021–1035.

Haeberle EJ. The sex atlas—a new illustrated guide. New York: Seabury Press, 1978: 7–59.

Holmes KK, Mardh PA, Sparling PF, Weisner PJ. Sexually transmitted diseases. New York: McGraw-Hill, 1984: 145–161, 161–173.

Masters WH, Johnson VE. Human sexual inadequacy. Boston: Little, Brown and Co, 1970: 85–91.

Masters WH, Johnson VE. Human sexual responses. London: Churchill, 1966: 27–82, 111–126, 171–220.

CONTRACEPTION

Adolescent Contraception

Each year in the United States, 1.3 million adolescents become pregnant. In Canada, an estimated 40,000 teenagers become pregnant. More than 500,000 of these elect to terminate their pregnancies, representing one-third of all legal abortions. Of those who carry their pregnancies to term, fewer than 7 percent give up their babies for adoption.

At puberty, adolescents must learn to cope with physical changes and complex psychological developments. In a few short years they develop secondary sex characteristics and reproductive capacity. They also establish their feminine or masculine personas.

Adolescence is often an awkward period for communication between doctor and patient, parent and child, teacher and student. Thus, sexual matters are often poorly dealt with.

First menstruation, or menarche, in North American women occurs at a mean age of 12.7 years, plus or minus 1.2 years. It is advisable for young adolescents to be taught, prior to menarche, about menstruation, development of secondary sexual characteristics and pregnancy.

Initially, menstruation can be expected to be painless and often irregular until a pattern of ovulation becomes established. The maturation of the hormonal cycle, with its regularly spaced ovulations and menstruations, may take months or years to achieve.

Adolescents who first report painless menstruations, later followed by premenstrual symptoms and menstrual discomfort, should be reassured that such changes are normal and represent the establishment of ovulatory, release-of-the-egg, cycles. Pain on menstruation, or dysmenorrhea, is normal for many, caused by the production of substances called prostaglandins.

Teachers and students are reminded that adolescents cannot rely on regular predictable ovulations. They are apt to have more spontaneous ovulations than older women and should not engage in unprotected intercourse at any time during their cycle, including during menstrual flow.

In fact, it is possible for any female to become pregnant at any time during the menstrual cycle. Even if ovulations are predictable, they may spontaneously occur on any given day.

Even though missed periods are normal for adolescents, this may be a sign of pregnancy if the female is sexually active. In such an instance, she should seek medical care to deal with pregnancy or as an opportunity to learn about contraceptive means.

The decrease in average age of menarche means that some females can conceive at a younger age. It is not surprising that those adolescents with adult reproductive capabilities have a "sex drive." They face the awesome task, at a very young age, of developing their own sexual identities as well as personal values about sexual behavior. At this level of adolescent development, parents, teachers and doctors should form a network to ensure proper guidance for the young. Sexual counseling should include education of the facts. counselors should help adolescents to help themselves to decide whether they are ready for sexual intimacy and prepared to assume the responsibility for their sexual behavior.

Too often parents do not have adequate information with which to educate their children. The majority have little knowledge of human physiology. In these cases, the responsibility for their children's education should be extended to specially trained counselors or teachers and physicians. Parents also often find it awkward to talk about sexual matters with their teenagers; still others feel that talking about sex is tantamount to issuing a license to have sex.

Adolescents can be kept ignorant of the facts—they cannot be kept from developing sexually or having sexual drives. They are entitled to objective unbiased advice. They should also be instructed as to what is acceptable and responsible sexual behavior.

The counselor and teacher's task in sexual education should be to pick up where parents leave off. And so it is necessary for parents to realize they have a most important role in counseling their children. Adolescents who have received some guidance from their parents on contraception are more apt to consistently use contraceptives.

A teenager's first enquiries are often directed at a physician. A teenage girl may wish to have a prescription for the birth control pill or to be fitted for a diaphragm. These patients should be reassured that they will benefit from the same confidentiality as do adults, that what transpires between an adolescent patient and his or her doctor will remain private.

This approach to teenage contraception and sexual counseling will anger some parents, who feel a doctor has no right to prescribe contraceptives to their children without their consent. These parents should be reminded that a prescription for contraceptives is based on an evaluation of medical needs, and it is preferable to instruct and prescribe in order to avoid an unwanted pregnancy or an abortion. Eighty-five percent of adolescents asking for contraceptives are already sexually active; therefore, education and the prescribing of contraceptives cannot be viewed as encouraging sexual activity in teenagers.

In 1972 the American Medical Association recommended that:

> The teenage girl whose sexual behavior exposes her to possible conception has access to medical consultation and the most effective contraceptive advice and methods consistent with her physical and emotional needs; and the physician so consulted should be free to prescribe or withhold contraceptive advice in accordance with his best medical judgment in the best interests of his patient.

As stated earlier, sexually active women between 15 and 19 years of age account for one-third of legal abortions. Few teenagers fail to use contraception because they want to get pregnant. Most enter into intimate relationships with too little knowledge and/or too many misconceptions. Reasons given for accidental pregnancies in this age group include:

1. Belief that they are too young to become pregnant
2. That they have intercourse too infrequently to become pregnant
3. That they have intercourse at a safe time of the month
4. That they did not expect to have intercourse
5. That early withdrawal of the male penis prior to ejaculation prevents pregnancy

Surveys indicate that many adolescents use contraceptive methods, sporadically or not at all, for as long as one year. One half of initial premarital teenage pregnancies occur in the first six months of sexual activity. Despite the rapid diffusion of modern contraceptive practices among unmarried, sexually active teenagers, pregnancy rates in this population have not changed.

Zelnick and Kantner (1976) report reasons for non-use in pregnant teenagers between 15–19 as follows:

1.	Didn't expect to have intercourse	43.0%
2.	Wanted to use something but under the circumstances was unable	10.1%
3.	Partner objected	9.3%
4.	Believed it was wrong or dangerous to use contraception	12.5%
5.	Did not know about contraception or where to get it	3.5%
6.	Contraception too difficult to use or sex not much fun with contraception	7.1%

Only 3.5 percent of pregnant teenagers did not know about contraception or where to get it. Access to protective measures does not seem to be of major importance, but rather, sporadic unexpected sexual encounters seem to preclude planned protection.

Many adolescents who establish intimate relationships with members of the opposite sex do not appear to recognize contraception as a major factor in healthy sexual functioning. They seem unable to relate to their own sex drive and have no vision of things to come.

Of those 4 percent of teenagers who had intercourse only once but did not want to become pregnant, 65 percent believed that because intercourse took place during a "safe" time of the month, they could not become pregnant. It would seem, then, that misinformation, combined with impulsive behavior, leads to failure to practice contraception.

Adolescent pregnancy resulting from non-use of contraception is not adequately handled by the family planning services or sex education in schools. Not enough teenagers are getting information or services needed prior to first sexual encounters. Only by providing such services will we be able to reduce the number of unwanted pregnancies and abortions in this age group.

Any effective program should take into account: increasingly early first sexual experiences of teenagers, the unplanned and sporadic nature of many such sexual encounters and ignorance about risk of pregnancy.

Many new educational methods are being developed; the most accepted means appear to involve small group discussions. Information should be detailed on all types of contraception: what each type is, how it is used, its effectiveness and associated risks. Myths that teenagers have about pregnancy must be dispelled, and they must be taught to accept responsibility for their sexual behavior. Early pregnancy is best prevented through primary prevention.

One education model uses a ''cognitive-behavioral approach'' to prevent pregnancy, as described by Schinke at the University of Washington. Specifically, this combines teaching factual information about human reproduction and contraception, as well as developing problem-solving abilities as they pertain to birth control. ''Responsible sexual behavior involves interpersonal communication so that young people can obtain contraception, regulate sexual encounters, and negotiate the use of birth control,'' as Schinke, in 1981, has noted.

Classes set up use small groups. The model described consists of fourteen 50-minute sessions. Topics covered are reproductive biology and contraceptive methods. Modalities used include guest speakers, audiovisual aids and open discussion. Information sessions are followed by problem solving, which deals with specific concerns, coming up with ways of handling those concerns, judging the worth and payoffs of these options and planning how to apply selected options in demand situations, i.e., unexpected moment of passion. Areas explored include dating, sexuality, birth control, pregnancy, abortion, child bearing and parenthood. Verbal and non-verbal communication are taught through role playing, modeling, acting out according to instructions, and rehearsal.

Teenagers with whom the above approach has been used have become more favorably disposed to family planning. They practice more effective birth control than those who are taught only via more conventional methods.

Adult Contraception

Problems relating to contraceptive practices of adults are seemingly more complex than those pertaining to teenagers. (See Figure 3-1 for the effectiveness of various birth control methods.) Several factors will be examined that may explain the still high number of unwanted pregnancies. For adults contraception is widely available, information accessible, and sexual activity outside marriage accepted by most. And yet still on university and college campuses everywhere, young adults are poor contraceptive users. One problem in being able to influence this group is that once out of secondary school systems these people are not readily accessible for teaching and counseling.

First-year college or university serves as an initiation to sex for up to 50 percent of students. Statistics show that women are as sexually active as men. No longer do we see the double standard of men outnumbering women two to one in this regard.

Increasingly, men and women also find sex to be acceptable within a brief relationship. As casual relationships become more commonplace, so too their inevitable consequences, sexually transmitted diseases. Fortunately, the majority of young adults still report a small number of sexual partners—only five percent have ten or more—and relationships are usually based on mutual understanding and closeness.

As with young adolescents, there are a large number of young adults who fail to use contraception at the time of their first intercourse, or they use unreliable methods—withdrawal, rhythm or douching. Prevalence figures for this group range from 52 to 76 percent, indicating that a majority is at risk at this time. Contraceptive use does become much more prevalent with subsequent encounters; 28 to 40 percent report unreliable methods or no method used.

Couples living together report non-use at 12 percent and unreliable use at 0 percent, whereas casual encounters report non-use at 36 percent and unreliable use at 6 percent.

We can conclude that contraceptive use improves with sexual experience and age and is most often practiced within a committed relationship.

When contraception is practiced in first sexual encounters among university-aged students, the condom is used most frequently by 19 to 40 percent of couples. Oral contraceptive use at first intercourse is measured at only 2 to 12 percent, as compared to 76 percent for sexually active adult women.

Recently there has been an increase in the use of condoms because women are more concerned about the possible side effects of the birth control pill and are aware of the role of condoms and spermicidal gels in preventing the spread of sexually transmitted diseases.

It is generally accepted that 5 to 10 percent of college or university students get pregnant each year, and that 16 percent of sexually active students have had at least one abortion.

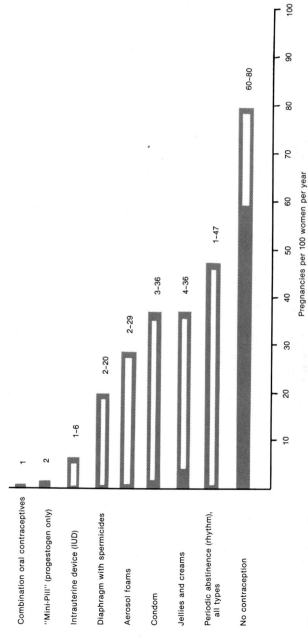

Figure 3–1 The effectiveness of various birth control methods. The figures (except for oral contraceptives and the IUD) vary widely because people differ in how well they use each method. Very faithful users of the various methods may achieve pregnancy rates in the lower ranges. Other women may expect pregnancy rates more in the middle of these ranges.

Ninety percent of student pregnancies are aborted.

The degree of contraceptive knowledge is not a good predictor of contraceptive use, even in adults. Certainly some young adults may still have misconceptions or be misinformed, but it appears that other factors play a role in poor contraceptive practices.

A study done at Rutger University found that for a woman to be motivated to use a contraceptive method effectively and efficiently, she must be satisfied with the aesthetic properties of her method, its efficiency, and its safety. One presumes the same would be true of men practicing contraception. Counseling, then, should be frank but should also emphasize the positive aspects of contraceptive methods discussed.

The Guilt Theory

According to some researchers, one reason for failure to use proper contraceptive measures has been the belief that sexual knowledge and preparedness mean a loss of innocence, a reflection of oneself as a sexual being. This applies mostly to women. In order to be prepared they must acknowledge their own sexuality, deal with residues of the old double standard—which holds that it is acceptable for men to be sexually active but not for women—and face the fear of being rejected by a partner for being "promiscuous." This guilt complex leads to denial and acting as if sex were not going to occur. These feelings lead to behavior that inhibits contraceptive use.

Byrne and his followers have labelled such people "erotophobes." He feels that a non-anxious society that is sexually free would only produce "erotophiles," whose sexual behavior would be characterized by responsible contraceptive behavior.

Erotophobia will inhibit proper contraceptive use in a number of ways:

Planning to have sex. Sexual intent would be anxiety provoking. Anxiety can be allayed by having "spontaneous sex," i.e., under the influence of alcohol, drugs or passion.

Obtaining contraceptive devices. Publicly acknowledging one's intention by acquiring contraceptive devices from a doctor or a druggist is felt to cause negative perceptions of his or her sexual being, further inhibiting contraceptive use.

Communication between partners about contraception. Discussion of sexual intercourse is awkward for the erotophobe and is often delayed or completely ignored.

Using the contraceptive device or technique. This is a reminder that the sexual act is for pleasure, not for reproduction, causing anxiety in the erotophobe. Such contraceptive practices may involve genital contact, and this may be difficult for the erotophobem, who associates touching his or her genitals with shame or dirtiness.

Testing revealed that those who score as erotophobic have difficulty talking about sex, acquiring contraceptive devices and are, on the whole, poor contraceptive users. Erotophiles, on the other hand, are more likely to go to family planning clinics, discuss contraception with parents, teachers or doctors. They are more comfortable with coitus-dependent methods, the condom, diaphragm and spermicides. They have a positive perception of sex. According to Lief, educational programs might, therefore, involve a process of "desensitization," whereby an individual becomes less anxious and embarrassed by sexual matters. Then, through "sensitization," he or she develops a greater awareness of his or her feelings about sex. And finally, through a process of integration, the person incorporates new knowledge about sexuality into his or her new attitude.

Another important research group, Mosher and his associates, also found that guilt has an inhibiting effect on proper contraceptive use. In turn, the theories of Byrne and Mosher reinforce the notion that the immediate psychic risks of being prepared far outweigh the distant risk of getting pregnant.

By contrast to the problem posed by erotophobia, in committed relationships, individuals are able to rid themselves of guilt; the fact of being in love or being committed to one person makes having sex acceptable.

Self-esteem

A recurrent theme among such researchers as Zelnick and Kautner, Lindeman, Bradwick and others, is that of self-esteem and/or feelings of personal powerfulness through the use of effective contraception. This can also be expressed as the ability to consciously try to sort out contraceptive issues or to feel comfortable with the idea of premeditated sex, i.e., contraceptive responsibilty without negative psychological sequelae.

This feeling of self-worth enables one to see beyond the immediate gratification of sexual urges and attach more importance to risks of unprotected intercourse.

Sex-role Attitudes

Non-traditional attitudes towards the female role, such as equality with men and career orientation, indirectly contribute to the effective use of contraceptives in young adults. The traditional view, or sex-role perception, is that some young women do not use contraceptives because they adhere to such traditional attitudes. They may be part of a career-oriented group yet, consciously or unconsciously, they desire pregnancy and do not contracept properly or at all. For those women who consciously wish for equal status with men, the non-traditional role, contraception is more effective.

Sex-role attitudes are also directly involved in contraception. A woman often assumes complete responsibility for contraception, unable to involve the man in what he may consider to be a nuisance or a "turnoff." She, in order not to disturb her partner's pleasure, will undertake to inform herself, acquire and use contraceptives. A non-traditional woman, on the other hand, will solicit her partner's input and involvement and is more likely to require that he join her in contraceptive decision making, insist that he wear a condom, or that he pay for birth control pills. It is quite likely that this woman's ability to contracept will be adequate, as she places her security above his pleasure.

Similar changes in attitudes are occurring in men who are not threatened by a woman's changing role and who recognize their role in contraception. In campus health services it is now common to see men and women inquiring together about contraception, and even to see men coming in alone for contraception counseling, eager to do their share.

Education

So how can we best deal with the overwhelming facts that:

1. First coital experiences are marked by poor contraceptive protection
2. That young people deny sex as an anticipated act and therefore excuse their actions with the claim that they were caught up in a moment of passion and were, therefore, not responsible
3. That poor knowledge of contraception is associated with higher pregnancy rates
4. Poor self-esteem and traditional attitudes towards sex are also linked with failure to contracept?

The answer seems obvious. Educational programs have to be set up early, when reproductive capabilities are developing. Programs for university and college students would differ from those for adolescents. The latter group requires factual knowledge and problem-solving development, while the former requires more than information. Programs should incorporate the idea that contraception for many is primarily sexual. According to Byrne, counselors should emphasize emotion in the act itself, help lessen guilt and anxiety, and increase comfort with sex as a natural human function.

The reader may believe that talking about sexual matters will only encourage adolescents to explore their desires. Proper education, if it did not discourage sexual encounters in adolescents, would at least decrease the likelihood of unwanted pregnancies or sexually transmitted disease.

If we can impart knowledge to the people, we can also affect behavior. Educational programs can also delay premature sexual encounters by emphasizing timing of intercourse and favorable conditions, acceptable behavior and responsibility. More teenagers might be prepared to admit they are not ready for sex or for intimate sexual relationships. Those who feel prepared would be armed with sufficient knowledge to avoid complications.

In the following section, currently accepted methods of contraception will be listed, and the pros and cons of each will be discussed. The method of contraception you choose must satisfy these criteria in the following areas:

1. **Safety**.   Most methods of contraception available today have very high safety levels. You should be aware, however, that the degree of safety is influenced by the risks of failure, i.e., having an unwanted pregnancy, that are present in a given technique.
2. **Effectiveness**.   You should be familiar not only with the lowest failure rates observed among carefully instructed and highly motivated people, but also with rates which apply to typical users in everyday life.
3. **Ease of use and acceptibility**.   Any method, to be effective, must be used properly every time intercourse takes place.

Further Reading

Bachmann GA. Model for effective contraceptive counseling on campus. College Health 1981; 30:119–121.

Byrne D, Jazwinski C, DeNinno J, Fisher W. Negative sexual attitudes and contraception. In: Byrne D, Byrne LA, eds. Exploring human sexuality. New York: Harper and Row, 1977.

Fox GL. Sex-role attitudes as predictors of contraceptive use among unmarried university students. Sex Roles 1977; 3:265–283.

Gold D, Berger C. The influence of psychological and situational factors on the contraceptive behaviour of single men: a review of the literature. Popul Environ 1983; 6:113–129.

Keller JF, Sack AR. Sex guilt and the use of contraception among unmarried women. Contraception 1982; 25:388–393.

Lief H. Obstacles to the ideal and complete sex education of the medical student and physician. In: Zubin J, Money J, eds. Contemporary sexual behavior: critical issues in the 1970s. New York: Bantam Books, 1975.

Mosher DL. Measurement of guilt in females by self-report inventories. J Clin Psychol 1968; 32:690–695.

Reading AE, Cox DN, Sledmere CM. Psychological issues arising from the development of new male contraceptive. Bull Br Psychol Soc 1982; 35:360–371.

Rindskopf KD. A perilous paradox: the contraceptive behavior of college students. College Health 1981; 30:113–118.

Schinke SP, Blythe BJ, Gilchrist LD. Cognitive-behavioral prevention of adolescent pregnancy. J Counsel Psychol 1981; 28:451–454.

Zelnick M, Kantner JF. Reasons for nonuse of contraception by sexually active women aged 15–19. Fam Plann Perspect 1979; 11:289–296.

HORMONAL CONTRACEPTION

Birth Control Pill

The birth control pill, currently the most effective reversible method of contraception, was introduced to the North American market in the early 1960s. Its use increased rapidly until the mid 1970s, when reports in the lay press of complications precipitated a return to other, more "natural" forms of birth control. However, the facts were often distorted, and important information was left out.

Since the first combination of estrogen and progesterone was marketed, several generations of "the pill" have been developed in an attempt to minimize side effects while maintaining efficacy. The lower-dose contraceptives now on the market contain approximately one-fifth the original estrogen content and one-twentieth the progesterone. This may explain why, although the list of the pill's reported side effects is extensive, the incidence of adverse reactions has been drastically reduced.

Another recent achievement is the development of the biphasic and triphasic oral contraceptive. With the traditional pill, a woman would ingest the same combination of hormones throughout her menstrual cycle. In an attempt to more closely simulate female physiology, several pharmaceutical companies manufacture a product whose dose schedule closely follows the hormonal changes that occur during the menstrual cycle. This has allowed a further reduction in the incidence of side effects and a decrease in the total hormone dose during one cycle.

After oral contraceptives became available, and various complications highlighted, epidemiological studies were undertaken to define these complications and determine the contributing risk factors. Now, more than twenty years later, clear criteria provide for careful screening and follow-up of pill users, so that women at low risk can feel comfortable taking this method of birth control.

Mechanism of Action

Combination-type birth control pills contain both estrogen and progesterone, two hormones produced naturally by the ovaries. They prevent pregnancy by acting both centrally and peripherally to inhibit ovulation (Fig. 4-1) and to interfere with the normal transport of sperm. Ovulation is inhibited by the suppression of gonadotrophin release, that is, LH and FSH. With the presence of hormones from the pill, the brain is led to be-

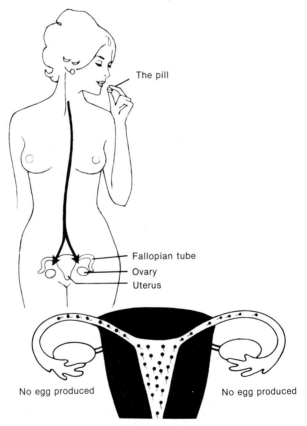

The pill

Fallopian tube
Ovary
Uterus

No egg produced   No egg produced

Figure 4–1 Mechanism of action of birth control pill: oral contraceptives prevent the production of eggs by a negative feedback mechanism. (Reproduced with permission by Wyeth Ltd.)

lieve the ovaries are producing enough hormone; thus, by a feed-back mechanism, the pituitary gland controls any further release of LH and FSH. Without the stimulating effect of these gonadotrophins, maturation of the ovum and ovulation cannot occur.

A similar feedback mechanism prevents ovulation in pregnancy, since the developing fetus and its placenta have a comparable inhibiting effect on gonadotrophin release.

When the birth control pill is taken properly, the incidence of ovulation is less than 2 percent. Even in the face of an "escaped" ovulation, the pill continues to exercise its contraceptive effect. Progestin, progesterone, causes changes that make fertilization of the ovum and implantation, imbedding of developing egg into the wall of the uterus, more difficult. Cervical mucus becomes thick and impenetrable to sperm, and transport of sperm and egg becomes more difficult, as well.

Efficiency

The lowest observed failure rate for the birth control pill is 0.5 percent; the failure rate in typical users is closer to 2 percent. Maximum efficiency is achieved when the pill is taken properly, that is to say, for 21 consecutive days followed by a seven day rest period. In the case of 28-day paquets, during the seven day rest period, sugar pills, placebos, are taken in order to encourage the habit of taking one pill every day. This cyclical use of the pill is equally effective whether a woman's natural cycle is 25 or 33 days, or completely irregular.

Pros

1. Most effective method
2. Causes lighter menstrual flow, resulting in decreased incidence of anemia
3. Does not interfere with sexual activity or spontaneity
4. Promotes very regular cycles
5. Decreases premenstrual tension
6. Decreases dysmenorrhea (painful menstruation)
7. Provides some protection against: benign breast disease; pelvic inflammatory disease caused by gonorrhea, a major cause of infertility; rheumatoid arthritis; cancer of the endometrium, the lining of the uterus; ovarian cancer (Fig. 4-2A, 2B)
8. May improve acne

Cons

1. One pill must be taken each day
2. Cannot be used while breast feeding

A

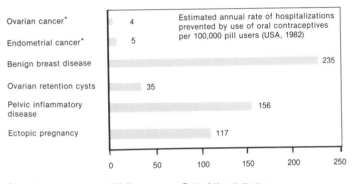

Ovarian cancer*

Endometrial cancer*

Benign breast disease

Ovarian retention cysts

Pelvic inflammatory disease

Ectopic pregnancy

*Based on ever-users aged 20–54   Rate of Hospitalizations

B

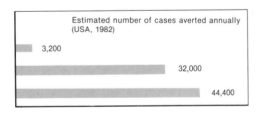

Rheumatoid arthritis

Iron-deficiency anemia

Pelvic inflammatory disease

Figure 4–2 *A*, Reduced hospitalization rates for a number of clinical conditions have been demonstrated recently in the United States. *B*, The use of oral contraceptives also prevents a number of diseases that usually do not require hospitalization.

Side Effects

The use of increasingly lower dosages of both estrogen and progestogen in newer formulations of the pill has reduced the risks and side effects to a consistently low level.

In prescribing birth control pills, physicians try to obtain for their patients the lowest possible dosage. These low-dosage combination pills are just as effective in preventing pregnancy as their higher-dosage counterparts. Occasionally, hormonal requirements of a given patient will not be met by these pills, even though contraception is assured. In such cases medium-range pills may be necessary to obtain a regular cycle with acceptable menstrual flow.

When a patient complains of a given side effect, it may be possible simply to change to another pill—often in the same dosage range. Such side effects will usually disappear.

Most women will not experience any of the following side effects:

Predisposition to vaginitis.   Women on the pill have an altered vaginal pH. This change in acidity of the vagina may create a favorable environment for growth of benign but troublesome fungal organisms, especially *Candida albicans*. These can be controlled with vaginal creams. Some control can be obtained as well, by avoiding vaginal douches, perfumed tampons or the use of one tampon for a long period of time, by wearing cotton undergarments rather than synthetic and by avoiding tight-fitting jeans. Symptoms of vaginal infection should be reported to a physician, so that appropriate cultures may be taken and treatment administered.

Pill users may also note a change in vaginal secretions that are not related to infection. These secretions usually appear normal in character but increase in quantity. There are no other related symptoms, however.

Headaches.   One-third of those women already suffering from headaches, especially migraines, may see a worsening of their headaches and an increase in frequency. They may need to discontinue the pill or switch to one of lower estrogen content.

Depression.   Depression or mood changes affect approximately 5 percent of pill users. Often this symptom can be corrected with vitamin B supplements, or through the use of a lower dosage pill.

Fluid retention and weight gain.   Oral contraceptives may have this effect. Progesterone may influence general weight gain, while estrogen may cause fluid retention and fat gain to breasts, thighs, and hips. These effects can be minimized by using low-dosage preparations.

Break-through bleeding. A common complaint in women using low-dosage pills is the occurrence of vaginal bleeding other than during menstruation. This is called "spotting," or break-through bleeding. It is directly related to low-estrogen content and can be corrected by switching to a higher estrogen level or to a pill whose progestin has higher endometrial activity, in other words, can cause adequate development of the inner lining of uterus.

Absence of menstrual flow. Again with low estrogen content, poor development of the inner lining of the uterus, the endometrium, will cause diminished menstrual flow. This is a desired effect. However, if flow stops altogether, the user and physician may consider the possibility of pregnancy. If break-through bleeding does not occur and if pregnancy tests are negative, the user need not even change the oral contraceptive.

Breast pain or tenderness. This is secondary to fluid retention and is easily corrected by decreasing estrogen content or increasing the progesterone fraction.

Visual changes. Women who wear contact lenses may notice changes in their visual acuity. This is caused by fluid retention in the cornea. Again this effect is rare in low-dosage estrogen pills and is completely reversible.

Acne and hair increase or decrease. Acne and hair growth, either facial or on the breasts, are caused by the androgenic, or masculinization, effect of testosterone. Normally, the adrenal glands and the ovaries produce small quantities of this hormone in women. Just as oral contraceptives work by suppressing ovarian function, so are the androgens, normally produced by the ovaries, suppressed. Therefore, while on the pill, most women will find conditions of acne and undesired facial and body hair improve.

In the minority of women who are sensitive to the androgenic effect of the pill itself, acne and hair growth will be minimized if the oral contraceptive is changed to a higher estrogen dosage.

Chloasma. Chloasma, or mask of pregnancy, describes a phenomenon of unknown cause, whereby pregnant women, and occasionally women on the pill, will develop brown patches of irregular shape over the face. They are usually barely noticeable. Those women with dark complexions or who expose themselves excessively to the sun seem most affected. Again, symptoms improve if these women are switched to lower estrogen-content oral contraceptives.

Nausea.   Nausea of pregnancy and nausea of the birth control pill are quite similar. The condition usually improves with time and is less noticeable if the pill is taken at bedtime with food. If nausea continues after three to four months use of the pill, a decrease in estrogen content is advisable.

Contraindications

Before the birth control pill can be prescribed, a complete history and physical examination are required. If the woman has not yet had sexual intercourse, the vaginal exam and PAP test may be delayed until sexual intercourse has taken place.

Women who are at greater risk of suffering adverse reactions or complications will be screened out at this time, and an alternate method of contraception suggested to them.

Even adolescents who have only recently started menstruating may safely use the pill for contraception. There is no evidence that the pill harms future reproductive capabilities if menstrual cycles have already begun. Nor are growth patterns altered by the introduction of the pill.

Contraindications, instances when you should not be taking the pill, are briefly reviewed.

Absolute Contraindications

Pregnancy.   The birth control pill should not be started until it is clear a woman is not already pregnant. One way of determining this is to ensure that a woman starts the pill only after she has had a normal menstruation.

If the pill is taken during pregnancy, menstruation may occur, and pregnancy will not be suspected until after it is well established. Children born to women who have taken the pill early in pregnancy are usually normal, but a higher incidence of congenital problems has been reported.

History of hypertension, heart disease, thrombophlebitis.   Those women who suffer or have suffered from any of the above should choose an alternate method of contraception. They fall into a high risk group for future complications.

Undiagnosed, abnormal genital bleeding. Women who have gynecological disorders that have not been diagnosed, should find the cause before taking oral contraceptives.

Impaired liver function and jaundice of pregnancy. Women with liver impairment should not use oral contraceptives. Those who have suffered from hepatitis of viral origin, but whose liver function has been completely restored, may safely use the pill.

Known or suspected cancer of the breast. Among pill users, many studies have shown a reduction in total incidence of benign or fibrocystic breast disease and a lower rate of breast cancer. Yet, it appears that those women with cancer of the breast at the time of starting oral contraceptives, may experience an increase in tumor size.

Women with strong family histories of breast cancer, and those who have breast nodules or fibrocystic disease, should have careful follow-up if they choose to use oral contraceptives.

Known or suspected estrogen dependent cancer. Some cancers grow more rapidly when exposed to estrogens. A patient with a history of having had cancer in the past should consult her physician regarding the safety of oral contraceptives for her.

Relative Contraindications

In these instances it may be preferable to use oral contraceptives only if an acceptable efficient alternative cannot be found.

Migraine headaches. One-third of migraine sufferers will experience a greater number of headaches, as well as an increase in their severity.

Hypertension. Even though blood pressure can still be managed while a woman is taking oral contraceptives, it is preferable to avoid the pill.

Fibroids. These may enlarge under the influence of estrogen. If the pill is used, low-dosage estrogen preparations are advised.

Epilepsy. It is possible that epilepsy may be more difficult to control in conjunction with oral contraceptive use. Women taking medication to control seizures may also be exposed to a drug interaction that could diminish the efficiency of the oral contraceptive.

Varicose veins. These may worsen, further predisposing a woman to possible phlebitis associated with pill use.

Gestational diabetes. Women who develop diabetes in pregnancy may develop a similar problem while on oral contraceptives, especially if the preparation is a higher dosage.

Elective surgery. If a woman is to undergo a surgical procedure and be hospitalized for any length of time, she is at risk, as is anyone confined to bed, of developing phlebitis. Oral contraceptives at this time would only add to that risk.

Women over 35 years of age. Studies indicate that complications attributable to the birth control pill occur in women 35 years of age or more who smoke, or in women 45 years of age or more who do not smoke. In these cases an alternate method of contraception is wise.

When all is said and done, most women are ideal candidates for the birth control pill; fortunately, most young women are healthy. The use of increasingly lower dosages of estrogen and progesterone in newer formulations of the pill has reduced the incidence of risk factors and side effects to a very low level.

These risks and side effects must be weighed against the risks involved in pregnancy and take into account the beneficial effects of the pill on the menstrual cycle. The risk of death among teenagers using the pill is 1.3 per 100,000 users. This compares favorably to infant death rates of 11.1 per 100,000 live births. Considering the risk-benefit ratio, the use of low-dosage combined oral contraceptives is a safe, highly effective method of controlling fertility.

Serious Risks

Cardiovascular disease: thrombophlebitis, thrombosis, heart attacks, strokes

Venous Thrombosis and Venous Thrombophlebitis

Oral contraceptives used between 1960 and the mid 1970s were felt to be responsible for 19 cases of thromboembolic disease per 10,000 users per year. Mortality rates (Fig. 4-3A, 3B), in the absence of predisposing conditions, have been claculated at 1.3 per 1,000,000 users, in women between 20 and 34 years of age, and 3.4 per 100,000 users between the ages of 35 and 44. As there appears to be a direct correlation between estrogen and progestogen content and risk of overt venous

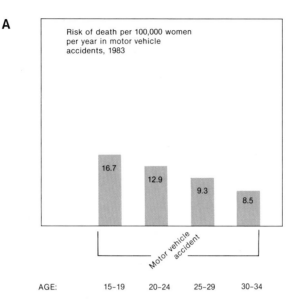

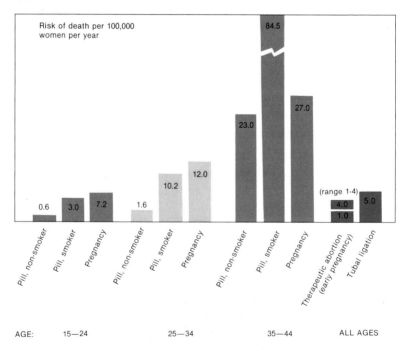

Figure 4-3 Risk of death in *A,* motor vehicle accidents, and *B,* risk of death in taking birth control pills compared to pregnancy, therapeutic abortions, and tubal ligation in various age groups.

thromboembolic disease, the condition would be less likely to occur with today's low-dosage pills.

When oral contraceptives are discontinued, risk of overt disease declines to the same level as for those women who have never used the pill.

Cigarette smoking and obesity probably do not play a significant role in the development of venous thromboembolic disease.

Myocardial Infarction (Heart Attack) and Stroke

The increased risk of myocardial infarction, or heart attack, among pill users appears to be unrelated to the duration of use, and the risk diminishes after the pill has been discontinued for one month. The risk among users between 25 and 49 years of age is three to four times that of those women who have never used oral contraceptives.

Similarly, the risk of thrombotic stroke among current users of oral contraceptives is increased.

Those factors that further increase the risk of myocardial infarction or strokes in pill users are: age greater than 35, cigarette smoking, history of hypertension or toxemia of pregnancy and diabetes.

Most of the risk is concentrated in women who are more than 35 years of age and in smokers who take oral contraceptives. The annual risk of death associated with pill use is as follows:

non-smokers:	1 per 100,000 women between 15 and 19 years of age to 3 per 100,000 women between 40 and 44.
smokers:	2 per 100,000 women between the ages of 15 and 19; 12 per 100,000 women 30 to 34 years of age; 61 per 100,000 women 40 to 44 years of age

However, these statistics are based on use of higher-dosage oral contraceptives than are generally prescribed today. With low-dose oral contraceptives the risk of cardiovascular disease, it is felt, has already been reduced.

In weighing the risks of the birth control pill, a physician must also consider pregnancy. In women under 35, the risk of death due to complications of pregnancy is about four to ten per 100,000, at least four times that related to oral contraceptive use.

Hypertension

Oral-contraceptive-induced hypertension, or high blood pressure, has been shown to be related to the length of use. It is also dose related and, therefore, unlikely to occur with low-dose pills. Once the pill has been discontinued, blood pressure returns to normal.

Liver Disorders

The incidence of gallbladder disorders, including gall stones, is twice as high among pill users in North American studies. British studies have not come up with the same relationships; still, oral contraceptives should be of low dosage to minimize this possibility.

Benign tumors of the liver are more common among oral contraceptive users; however, they are still very rare, one to two per 1,000,000 female users.

Myths

"The birth control pill causes cancer."

This is a myth. Oral contraceptives do *not* increase the risk of developing breast cancer; studies show no such pattern. In fact, women who have never used the pill often have more advanced tumors than those using oral contraceptives in the year prior to diagnosis of breast cancer. There is even evidence that oral contraceptives may protect for both the ovaries and the inner lining of the uterus, the endometrium, from such disease.

Oral contraceptive use in itself does not increase the risk of cervical cancer. Pill users, however, are more sexually active, and this is a well-known risk factor for cancer of the cervix. However, pill users are usually more closely monitored through annual pap smears, allowing for earlier detection.

"Every three or four years the pill should be discontinued
for a few months."

This is a myth. In the past, when much higher doses of hormones were used, a periodic return to normal cycles was deemed necessary. However, since our better understanding of ovulation has led to the introduction of combination pills in much lower doses, these brief interruptions in pill use will only increase the chances of unwanted pregnancy.

Also, since most recent studies have shown that there is no relationship between serious side effects and the duration of birth control pill use, there is no valid reason to discontinue oral contraceptives after ten years, as long as the patient's age is within acceptable limits and she remains healthy. Oral contraceptives are safe for healthy women up to 45 years of age if they are non-smokers, and for smokers who are no more than 35 years of age.

"Post-pill amenorrhea, lack of menstruation for six months to
one year, occurs after discontinuation of the pill."

This is a myth. The incidence of post-pill amenorrhea varies tremendously, according to different studies. Several other conditions might result in amenorrhea: body weight below the average for the population, obesity and preexisting menstrual irregularities. The pill will not impair long-term potential for pregnancy.

For patients who had regular menstrual cycles prior to taking the pill, spontaneous menstruation will usually resume within three months after stopping the pill. Those who do not see a return to normal cycles must be examined for possible pathological causes unrelated to the birth control pill.

"The pill may cause infertility."

This is a myth. When it is discontinued, previous fertility is reestablished. The pill's misleading association with infertility can be related to two factors. The first is that women who contracept well often choose to have children at a stage in their lives when there is a natural decline in fertility. If women were as fertile at the end of their reproductive lives as they are at the beginning, we would expect to find much larger families among our ancestors. Fortunately for them, reproductive capacity declines with age. It is not surprising then, to find that more and more women who decide to have their first child between the ages of 30 and 35 have more difficulty in becoming pregnant than younger women.

Further, though the birth control pill liberates many women, they then may expose themselves to more sexual partners, and more sexually transmitted diseases. This often leads to damage of the fallopian tubes and, ultimately, infertility.

"The pill will cause deformities in future children."

This is a myth. A slight increase in spontaneous abortion and birth defects has been purported to occur in pregnant women taking the pill. But there is absolutely no evidence that pregnancy, after discontinuation of oral contraceptives, involves any teratogenic, or deformity, risks.

In the United States, 8.4 million women use oral contraceptives at any given time. The net death rate for those taking birth control pills is 3.7 per 100,000 (nonsmokers, 1.8 ; smokers, 6.5) compared to a maternal mortality rate in the United States of 20.6 per 100,000 live births. Among those 8.4 million women, 310 deaths per year can be attributed to the pill. If those women clearly at risk did not use the pill, that number could be drastically reduced.

Oral contraceptives may offer the best combination of effectiveness and safety for women under the age of 35 who do not smoke and have no other risk factors. The degree of risk involved in taking low-dosage pills is virtually the same or lower than that of other methods, such as the intrauterine device, diaphragm or condom. It is ironic that in the past few years this same low-risk group has tended to use the birth control pill much less, bending to pressure from the lay press, which until recently has encouraged more natural, less efficient methods of birth control.

Oral contraceptive users who are smokers and who are more than 30 years of age, women over 45 who do not smoke and women at risk because of other medical conditions, run a risk 2.5 times higher than those women who do not use oral contraception. That ratio remains below the maternal mortality rate, representing those who die through pregnancy and childbirth; still, for women at higher risk, alternate contraceptive methods should be encouraged. A justifiable conclusion is that, considering the risk-benefit ratio, low-dosage-combined oral contraceptives are a safe and highly effective method of controlling fertility.

Instructions for Oral Contraceptive Use

Certain practical aspects of pill use should be discussed. Accidental pregnancies usually occur either because women run out of or discontinue their prescriptions, or because they forget to take two or more pills. Proper contraceptive practices are important.

Remember that protection lapses shortly after you discontinue the pill, and that an alternate method should be used the very next day.

The following are recommendations for the proper use of the birth control pill.

1. Unless your physician or the product monograph instructs you otherwise, you should take your first pill on the fifth day of your period. The only logic in assigning day five is that most patients will receive similar instruction, therefore causing less confusion. In fact, the pill can be started at any time between the first to the tenth day of the menstrual cycle. Some companies set up their paquets to start on a Sunday. That way the last pill of the cycle will be taken on a Saturday, and it is not likely that these women will ever be bothered with menstruation on the weekends for as long as they are taking oral contraceptives.

2. From then on you take one pill daily for three weeks, 21 days, then no pills for one week, 7 days. This means you will start every new pack on the same day of the week. This will apply for a 21-day pack. For the 28-day pack, you will take one pill daily, without stopping between packs.

3. For those using the 21-day pack, your period will usually come during the week when you are not taking pills. Women using the 28-day pack should get their period while taking the last seven pills (Fig. 4-4). You are still protected during this week.

4. Use foam and a condom during the first 2 weeks of your initial pill-taking cycle.

5. Develop a routine by taking your pill at the same time every day. If you miss one or two pills, take them as soon as you remember, even if it means taking two or three at a time. If you miss two or more, you should use another method of contraception, such as foam and a condom, until the next cycle begins. Continue to take one pill daily. Bleeding may occur for a few days.

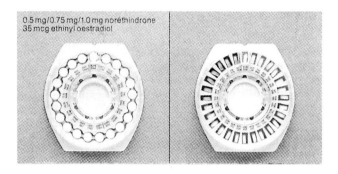

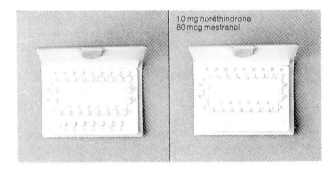

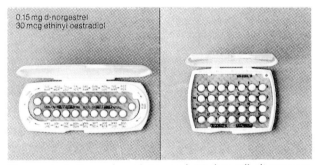

Figure 4–4 Examples of 21- and 28-day pill dispensers. (Courtesy of Syntex Laboratories Inc. and Ortho Pharmaceutical Corporation.)

6. Side effects may include nausea, breast enlargement, weight loss or gain, spotting or bleeding between periods, irritability and depression. Nausea can be alleviated by taking the pills before bedtime. Most side effects subside after one to three months.

7. Call your doctor if you experience depression, or any severe pain, blurring of vision, swelling of ankles or legs or increased crampiness in the legs.

8. Have an annual examination and pap smear or as advised by your doctor.

9. Return to the doctor in three months if you are taking the pill for the first time.

10. It is recommended that you quit smoking if you are taking oral contraceptives.

11. If you have spotting or bleeding while taking the first 21 pills of your paquet, continue on schedule, anyway. Symptoms will probably stop after three cycles. If they do not, see your physician. However, if bleeding is heavy, or if you experience bleeding and/or cramps or deep pelvic pain upon penetration of the penis, infection could be the cause. You should see your doctor as soon as possible.

12. Should you miss a menstrual period and you are sure you have taken your pills properly, don't worry; start your next pack. If, however, you have missed taking pills, you may be pregnant. STOP taking your pills. Use an alternate method of contraception and see your physician.

13. If you are ill and have been started on medication, remind your doctor that you are on the pill. Some medications interact with oral contraceptives to reduce the latter's efficiency. You may have to use another birth control method while following a prescribed treatment for another condition.

The pill can be stopped at any time during the cycle. Bleeding usually occurs two or three days after the last pill; this is your last "pill period." After that your body will reestablish its natural cycle.

In order to ensure the success of oral contraceptives, with minimal inconvenience, consider the following.

Reduce your pill risk. Cut down or stop smoking. If possible, stick to low-dosage pills (Table 4-1, 4-2). Have regular checkups, including PAP smears. If you are part of a high-risk group,

TABLE 4-1　Oral Contraceptives Available in Canada

Product	Manufacturer	Estrogen	μg/Tablet	Progestogen	μg/Tablet	mg. Total Hormonal Content/Cycle
			(days in brackets for biphasics & triphasics)			
20, 30 & 35 μg Estrogen—For conception control.						
Triphasil†‡	Wyeth	Ethinyl Estradiol	30(6),40(5),30(10)	d-Norgestrel§	50(6),75(5),125(10)	2.61
Min-Ovral	Wyeth	Ethinyl Estradiol	30	d-Norgestrel§	150	3.78
Minestrin 1/20	Parke-Davis	Ethinyl Estradiol	20	Norethindrone Acetate	1000	21.42
Loestrin 1.5/30	Parke-Davis	Ethinyl Estradiol	30	Norethindrone Acetate	1500	32.13
Demulen 30	Searle	Ethinyl Estradiol	30	Ethynodiol Diacetate	2000	42.63
Ortho 1/35	Ortho	Ethinyl Estradiol	35	Norethindrone	1000	21.74
Ortho 0.5/35	Ortho	Ethinyl Estradiol	35	Norethindrone	500	11.24
Brevicon 0.5/35	Syntex	Ethinyl Estradiol	35	Norethindrone	500	11.24
Brevicon 1/35	Syntex	Ethinyl Estradiol	35	Norethindrone	1000	21.74
Ortho 10/11‡#	Ortho	Ethinyl Estradiol	35(21)	Norethindrone	500(10),1000(11)	16.74
Ortho 7/7/7†‡	Ortho	Ethinyl Estradiol	35(21)	Norethindrone	500(7),750(7),1000(7)	16.49
50 μg Estrogen—For conception control only when lower dosage estrogen formulations prove to be unsatisfactory.						
Ovral	Wyeth	Ethinyl Estradiol	50	d-Norgestrel§	250	6.30
Norlestrin 1/50	Parke-Davis	Ethinyl Estradiol	50	Norethindrone Acetate	1000	22.05
Norlestrin 2.5/50	Parke-Davis	Ethinyl Estradiol	50	Norethindrone Acetate	2500	53.55
Demulen 50	Searle	Ethinyl Estradiol	50	Ethynodiol Diacetate	1000	22.05
Ortho-Novum 1/50	Ortho	Mestranol	50	Norethindrone	1000	22.05
Norinyl 1/50	Syntex	Mestranol	50	Norethindrone	1000	22.05

TABLE 4-1   Oral Contraceptives Available in Canada (Cont'd)

Product	Manufacturer	Estrogen	μg/Tablet	Progestogen	μg/Tablet	mg. Total Hormonal Content/Cycle
75 & 80 μg Estrogen—Should not be used for conception control.						
Enovid 5	Searle	Mestranol	75	Norethynodrel	5000	106.58
Ortho-Novum 5	Ortho	Mestranol	75	Norethindrone	5000	106.58
Ortho-Novum 1/80	Ortho	Mestranol	80	Norethindrone	1000	22.68
Norinyl 1/80	Syntex	Mestranol	80	Norethindrone	1000	22.68
100 μg Estrogen—Should not be used for conception control.						
Norinyl-2	Syntex	Mestranol	100	Norethindrone	2000	44.10
Enovid-E	Searle	Mestranol	100	Norethynodrel	2500	54.60
Ovulen 1	Searle	Mestranol	100	Ethynodiol Diacetate	1000	23.10
Ovulen 0.5	Searle	Mestranol	100	Ethynodiol Diacetate	500	12.60
Ortho-Novum 0.5	Ortho	Mestranol	100	Norethindrone	500	12.60
Ortho-Novum 2	Ortho	Mestranol	100	Norethindrone	2000	44.10
Estrogen Free						
Micronor	Ortho			Norethindrone	350	

* Most of the estrogen-progestogen combination products listed in this table are also available with inert tablets that permit uninterrupted 28-day cycles of therapy.
† Triphasic product.
‡ The number of days each dosage of estrogen and progestogen is to be taken is shown in brackets in the dosage columns.
§ Supplied as the dl-racemate in double the amount shown.
# Biphasic product.

Selection criteria

The lowest dosages of *both* ingredients that are consistent with the desired biological effects are the safest and best for your patient.

1. The recommended dosage of estrogen for contraception is 30–35 μg. Use the lowest dosage of any given progestogen that will provide for contraception and good cycle control.
2. OCs containing 50 μg of estrogen should be used only when good cycle control cannot be attained with compounds containing 30–35 μg of estrogen. Varying the dosage of the progestogen may aid in achieving good cycle control.
3. OCs containing less than 30 μg of estrogen may be associated with a higher incidence of breakthrough bleeding and spotting than that for the products containing 30 μg or more of estrogen.
4. The use of estrogen-progestogen combinations containing a daily dosage of estrogen in excess of 50 μg is not acceptable for contraception. These products may be given for other medical purposes and contraception may be an added benefit.

use another method of contraception. If you are 35 years of age or older, contemplate switching to an alternate method of contraception.

Develop a routine. Try to associate taking the pill with some other daily event, such as brushing your teeth, bedtime, breakfast, etc.—and be sure to check your pack to assure yourself that the previous day's pill was taken.

Remember pill danger signs. See your physician as soon as possible should they occur. These danger signs are easily remembered by thinking of the word "ACHES": A—Abdominal pain, severe; C—Chest pain or shortness of breath, severe; H—Headaches, usually severe; E—Eye problems like blurred vision, double vision, flashing lights, partial blindness; S—severe leg pain.

Remember annual check-ups. Some women will have to have follow-up visits more frequently, as advised by their physicians, for gynecological problems not related to the birth control pill. Regardless, do not let a prescription for contraceptives lapse and then find yourself unable to renew it.

Alteration in your pill cycle. If you wish to discontinue the pill or change the timing of your menstruation, contact your physician. For example, you may decide to practice another method of contraception until pregnancy is desired. Or you may choose to delay a menstruation that might inconvenience you during a vacation, sports competition, exams and the like. Your clinician can help you make proper decisions that will not hamper your contraception protection.

Mini Pills

Mini pills are oral contraceptives that contain only progestin—no estrogen; they have had limited use to date. Until studies are completed comparing them to the combined estrogen-progestin preparations already discussed, guidelines for their use will be the same as for those oral contraceptives containing estrogen.

Mini pills are usually reserved for women who should avoid estrogen preparations, for women who have increased headaches, high blood pressure or leg pain after taking combination pills and for women smokers who are 35 years of age and over. However, the mini pill is less effective than estrogen-progestogen pills and is associated with more frequent menstrual irregularity and spotting. It must be taken faithfully, since it is effective for only 24 hours, and it must be taken regularly, without the usual seven days off provided for with combination oral contraceptives.

Morning-after Pill

Women who have had intercourse without adequate protection often come to physicians afterwards in an effort to avoid unwanted pregnancies. Post-coital regimens, or so-called morning-after pills, may be prescribed within 24 to 72 hours of intercourse and they increase the likelihood of preventing pregnancy. Side effects associated with this method include irregular bleeding, nausea and vomiting.

There are various oral regimens in this group that can be used; a discussion of them is best left to each patient's physician. However, none of these post-coital methods presently practiced have been approved by the F.D.A or Canada Health and Welfare. They are, however, widely used. They have a failure rate of 0.3 to 0.6 percent. Still, they should not be relied on as acceptable contraceptive methods. When not effective, they are associated with a small increase in incidence of birth defects.

Consultation for post-coital contraception may be required if:

1. Unplanned intercourse has occurred and, therefore, no contraception was used.
2. The condom tore or slipped off, spilling sperm into the vagina.
3. Partners using the "rhythm" method did not properly calculate fertile days.
4. Diaphragm was improperly placed.
5. Vaginal spermicidal suppository did not dissolve.

The most common morning-after hormone treatment used in Canada is the birth control pill called Ovral. It is of intermediate strength, and dosages used for post-coital protection may cause side effects. Those women already at risk may be exposed to more serious complications than if they had been on low-dosage pills all along, or if pregnancy were to continue. Although small, the risk of teratogenic defects of the fetus is greater.

TABLE 4-2   Oral Contraceptives Available in the United States of America

Product	Manufacturer	Estrogen	μg/Tablet	Progestogen	μg/Tablet	mg. Total Hormonal Content/Cycle
50 Micrograms Estrogen						
Enovid 5 mg(20)	Searle	Mestranol	75	Norethynodrel	5000	101.50
Enovid-E(21)	Searle	Mestranol	100	Norethynodrel	2500	54.60
Norinyl 2 mg(20)	Syntex	Mestranol	100	Norethindrone	2000	42.00
Ortho-Novum 2 mg(21)	Ortho	Mestranol	100	Norethindrone	2000	44.10
Ovulen(21,28)	Searle	Mestranol	100	Ethynodiol Diacetate	1000	23.10
Norinyl 1+80(21,28)	Syntex	Mestranol	80	Norethindrone	1000	22.68
Ortho-Novum 1/80(21,28)	Ortho	Mestranol	80	Norethindrone	1000	22.68
50 Micrograms Estrogen						
Norlestrin 2.5/50(21,Fe)	Parke-Davis	Ethinyl Estradiol	50	Norethindrone Acetate	2500	53.55
Demulen(21,28)	Searle	Ethinyl Estradiol	50	Ethynodiol Diacetate	1000	22.05
Norinyl 1+50(21,28)	Syntex	Mestranol	50	Norethindrone	1000	22.05
Norlestrin 1/50(21,Fe)	Parke-Davis	Ethinyl Estradiol	50	Norethindrone Acetate	1000	22.05
Ortho-Novum 1/50(21,28)	Ortho	Mestranol	50	Norethindrone	1000	22.05
Ovcon-50(21,28)	Mead Johnson	Ethinyl Estradiol	50	Norethindrone	1000	22.05
Ovral(21,28)	Wyeth	Ethinyl Estradiol	50	Norgestrel	500	11.55
Sub-50 Micrograms Estrogen						
Loestrin 1.5/30(21,Fe)	Parke-Davis	Ethinyl Estradiol	30	Norethindrone Acetate	1500	32.13
Demulen 1/35(21,28)	Searle	Ethinyl Estradiol	35	Ethynodiol Diacetate	1000	21.73
Norinyl 1+35(21,28)	Syntex	Ethinyl Estradiol	35	Norethindrone	1000	21.73
Ortho-Novum 1/35(21,28)	Ortho	Ethinyl Estradiol	35	Norethindrone	1000	21.73
Ortho-Novum 10/11(21,28)	Ortho	Ethinyl Estradiol	35	Norethindrone	500	11.23(10)
(Modicon and O-N 1/35)					1000	21.73(11)
Loestrin 1/20(21,Fe)	Parke-Davis	Ethinyl Estradiol	20	Norethindrone Acetate	1000	21.42
Modicon(21,28)	Ortho	Ethinyl Estradiol	35	Norethindrone	500	11.23
Brevicon(21,28)	Syntex	Ethinyl Estradiol	35	Norethindrone	500	11.23
Ovcon-35(21,28)	Mead Johnson	Ethinyl Estradiol	35	Norethindrone	400	9.13
Lo/Ovral(21,28)	Wyeth	Ethinyl Estradiol	30	Norgestrel	300	6.93
Nordette(21,,28)	Wyeth	Ethinyl Estradiol	30	Levonorgestrel	150	3.78
Triphasil(21)	Wyeth	Ethinyl Estradiol	30(6),40(5),30(10)	d-Norgestrel	50(6),75(5),125(10)	2.61
Ortho 7/7/7	Ortho	Ethinyl Estradiol	35(21)	Norethindrone	500(7),750(7),1000(7)	16.49
Tri-Norinyl(21,28)	Syntex	Ethinyl Estradiol	35(21)	Norethindrone	500(7),1000(9),500(5)	15.73
Tri-Levlin	Berlex	Ethinyl Estradiol	30(6),40(5),30(10)	d-Norgestrel	50(6),75(5),125(10)	2.61

Days in brackets

Depo-Provera

The use of injectable progesterone, known as Depo-Provera, is still quite controversial. It can be administered by deep intramuscular injection once every 3 months for 150 mg of Depo-Provera, or once every 6 months for 300 mg of Depo- Provera. In those countries where it is used, it is recommended for women who should not take estrogen preparations, or for those who cannot take pills on a daily basis. Some underdeveloped countries have welcomed the preparation as a method to help control population growth.

Once the injection is given, the hormone is released slowly into the circulation. There is no opportunity to change your mind. Its major drawback is that for a period of six months to one year after discontinuing this contraceptive practice, a woman might not menstruate.

New methods of hormonal control are being developed but are not yet available commercially. These include:

Vaginal Ring

A plastic ring containing estrogen and progesterone would be inserted into the vagina, and the hormones liberated and absorbed through the vaginal wall into the blood stream. These hormones would act in the same manner as the birth control pill. After three weeks, the ring would be removed, allowing for menstruation, and the cycle would start over again after seven days.

Subcutaneous Implants

Small implants containing estrogen and progesterone would be injected under the skin. The hormones would be absorbed into the bloodstream to exert their contraceptive effect.

Birth Control Pill for Men

Research is being done to develop such a male oral contraceptive, but it will probably be another ten years before it becomes available. There is one major drawback to the male pill: female confidence. A recent study in the United States asked women if they would have intercourse while in their fertile period with men who said they were on oral contraceptives—80 percent said no. In other words, a woman wishing to avoid pregnancy would not depend on her partner's sense of repsonsibility. This method would only work well for committed couples.

Further Reading

Abramowicz M, ed. Oral contraceptives and the risk of cardiovascular disease. Med Lett 1983; 25:69–70.

Astedt B. Oral contraception and some debatable side effects. Acta Obstet Gynecol Scand [Suppl] 1982; 105:17–23.

Beck WW. Complications and contraindications of oral contraception. Clin Obstet Gynecol 1981; 24:893–901.

Bronson RA. Oral contraception: mechanism of action. Clin Obstet Gynecol 1981; 24:869–877.

Decherney AH. The use of birth control pills in women with medical disorders. Clin Obstet Gynecol 1981; 24:965–975.

Huppert LC. Vascular effects of hormonal contraception. Clin Obstet Gynecol 1981; 24:951–963.

Lucas WE. Estrogen—a cause of gynecologic cancer? Cancer 1981; 48:451–454.

Rosenfield A. The pill: an evaluation of recent studies. The Johns Hopkins Med J 1982; 150:177–180.

Shojania AM. Oral contraceptives: effects on folate and vitamin B12 metabolism. Can Med Assoc J 1982; 126:244–247.

Stadel BV. Oral contraceptives and cardiovascular disease: (part one). N Engl J Med 1981; 305:612–618.

Stadel BV. Oral contraceptives and cardiovascular disease: (part two). N Engl J Med 1981; 305:672–677.

Swan SH, Petitti DB. A review of problems of bias and confounding in epidemiologic studies of cervical neoplasia and oral contraceptive use. Am J Epidemiol 1982; 115:10–18.

Vessey M, Baron J, Doll R, McPherson K, Yeates D. Oral contraceptives and breast cancer: final report of an epidemiological study. Br J Cancer 1983; 47:455–462.

NATURAL FAMILY PLANNING

Methods in this group are also known collectively as the Fertility Awareness Method. They include the Billings Ovulation Method and the Symptothermal Method. These practices take advantage of the fact that women are at most times infertile throughout their reproductive lives. By identifying the fertile phase of the menstrual cycle using various parameters, intercourse is avoided around the period of ovulation. At other times intercourse can take place without much risk of conception. If sexual relations are desired during fertile days, suitable barrier methods can be used.

These methods are not recommended for those women who have irregular menstruations, that is, for those whose cycles vary by more than a few days from month to month. Users must also be highly motivated as careful charting is required, and both partners have to be prepared to abstain from sexual intercourse, or use barrier methods, or find other means of sexual gratification during fertile days.

In the first six to eight months of fertility awareness programs, it is wise to use some barrier method or the IUD until the users are absolutely sure of the woman's cycle, are comfortable with the method, and are able to keep consistent records.

The period of ovulation can be gauged in several ways:

Change in body temperature. A slight change in body temperature occurs immediately before and during ovulation. There is usually a slight drop followed by a small rise, indicating that ovulation has taken place. Body temperature is taken in the morning, preferably rectally. A chart is kept for several months to determine the time of ovulation.

Change in cervical mucus. Mucous discharge usually begins six days before ovulation. The increasing vaginal discharge, induced by the rising level of estrogen, indicates impending ovulation.

Calendar method.   If a woman has a regular cycle of 28 days, ovulation generally occurs 14 days prior to menstruation. A record of the menstrual cycle is kept for a period of 8 to 12 months, and the pattern recorded can be applied to predict the time of ovulation. If a woman's periods are irregular, it is much more difficult to determine the "safe" days. Illness and physical and emotional stresses, such as those that occur at exam time, can also disturb the menstrual cycle and upset calculation of the time of ovulation.

Physical symptoms.   Some women experience various symptoms, such as abdominal pain and breast tenderness, for example, at the time of ovulation.

Effectiveness.   Any or all of these means of determining the time of ovulation carry a 15 to 35 percent failure rate.

Pros.   Monitoring the body in these ways costs little or nothing and contributes to greater awareness of one's physiology.

Ovulation Method and Symptothermal Method

The Ovulation Method (OM) relies upon the observation and recording of changes in cervical mucus to identify the fertile phase of the menstrual cycle.

The Symptothermal Method (STM), involves all the measures described earlier, the observation and recording of: basal body temperature, cervical mucus changes, duration of six previous menstrual cycles and physical symptoms (Fig 5-1).

Randomized prospective studies of the use-effectiveness of the OM and STM methods show the STM to be superior to the OM at a ratio of two to one. In various studies, drop-out rates for both methods were quite high. More than one-half of those entering studies dropped out within one year. Most said they did so because of lack of interest or dissatisfaction with either method. Pregnancies in those who continue with these methods are usually due to inaccurate interpretation of mucous symptoms and failure to follow rules.

The World Health Organization found these methods to be ineffective in preventing pregnancy, based solely on its study of centres with experience in natural family planning. Still, in Columbia between 16 and 22 percent became pregnant within the first year; in five other countries, 19 percent overall became pregnant. Women from these centers had a 97 percent accuracy rate at predicting ovulation; only women with this rate of success took part in the effectiveness studies. Failure to contracept was due to couples knowingly taking chances.

While the effectiveness of the Ovulation Method, if used correctly, is theoretically 98.5 percent, failure to abstain from sex at the required time renders this method ineffective for general use. Only highly motivated couples who are committed to their method, and for whom pregnancy would not be a disaster, should use either the Ovulation or the Symptothermal Method of birth control.

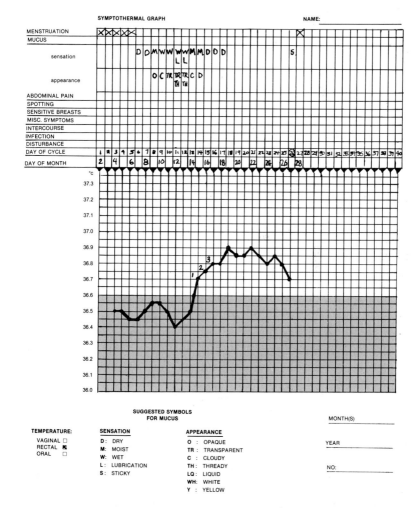

Figure 5–1 Symptothermal graph used to predict ovulation.

Pros

1. Eightly to 98 percent effective if implemented properly
2. Inexpensive
3. Safe
4. Contributes to greater awareness of female sexual physiology
5. When pregnancy is desired, can be used to predict fertility periods

Cons

1. Requires strong motivation on the part of both partners
2. High failure rate in practice, especially if menstrual cycles are irregular
3. Loss of spontaneity
4. Records must be kept for several months before these methods can be used
5. Often difficult to learn and time consuming to check body temperatures daily, as well as vaginal discharge

Physiological Principles of Natural Family Planning Methods

There are certain predictable events during each menstrual cycle. Yet, occasionally a cycle may be disrupted as the female body reacts to physical and/or emotional stress caused by disease, medication, dieting, weight gain, training, different life situations, etc. It is because of these possible irregularities that careful record keeping and strict adherence to the methodology are essential to guarantee the effectiveness of natural family planning.

Remember that six to eight cycles must be studied before a pattern of ovulation can be established.

Calendar Method

Records are kept of these half-dozen or more menstrual cycles. Day one is considered the first day of menstrual flow. In order to calculate the fertile period by this method, use the shortest cycle to find the first fertile day and the longest cycle to find the last fertile day.

Table 5–1 will be helpful:

Table 5-1   How to Calculate Your Fertile Period

Shortest Cycle	First Fertile Day	Longest Cycle	Last Fertile Day
21	3rd day	21	10th
22	4th	22	11th
23	5th	23	12th
24	6th	24	13th
25	7th	25	14th
26	8th	26	15th
27	9th	27	16th
28	10th	28	17th
29	11th	29	18th
30	12th	30	19th
31	13th	31	20th
32	14th	32	21st
33	15th	33	22nd
34	16th	34	23rd
35	17th	35	24th

day 1 = first day of menstrual bleeding
Reprinted from My Body, My Health. John Wiley and Sons, Inc.

According to the chart, if the shortest period is 25 days and the longest is 29, the unsafe time would be between the seventh and eighteenth days, inclusive. For all subsequent cycles, fertile days can be predicted by considering day one as the first day of menstrual flow.

Cervical Mucus

The observation of PEAK mucous symptoms closely correlates with the time of ovulation. In fact, such symptoms appear approximately six days prior to ovulation as an estrogen surge at this time stimulates the cervix. This mucus is needed for natural lubrication and to provide an ideal environment for conception.

At PEAK symptom time, cervical mucus is stretchy and lubricative. Mucous secretion is easily checked by inserting one or two fingers into the vagina and testing the consistency of the mucus by tapping finger and thumb together.

The most infertile days are those prior to ovulation, when mucus is relatively dry, and beyond the fourth day after ovulation, when mucus is tacky or pasty to dry. In the case of a short cycle of early ovulation, the PEAK symptoms have been observed even during menstrual flow, reinforcing the notion that conception can occur even during menstruation.

Women can learn to recognize changes in vaginal discharge. For most, in the days prior to ovulation, there will either be no discharge or sparse secretions. Women with "dry" days will notice the onset of transitional secretions that are thick and opaque before the PEAK symptom corresponding to ovulation, when secretions become more transparent and liquid, stretching as thread when examined and having a slippery lubricating texture. Women who normally secrete all through their cycle may find it difficult to assess a fertile pattern of secretion.

These changes were well studied and described by Drs. Evelyn and John Billings of Australia.

Mucus-method charts are kept, using letters to code observations made on various days. Unprotected intercourse should not take place from the first sign of mucus until the fourth night after the PEAK. On dry days, couples can have intercourse that night but not the next morning, as sperm remaining in the vaginal tract may be confused with the beginning of mucous production.

It must be stressed that vaginal secretion should be checked daily by putting a finger into the vagina and assessing how wet it feels. Any mucus collected should be then checked for stickiness and stretch, i.e. ability to form threads.

Some factors that may affect mucous readings include:

1. Vaginal infections
2. Intercourse the night before
3. Use of spermicidal preparations and lubricants
4. Douching
5. Medicated vaginal creams or suppositories

Basal Body Temperature Charting (BBT)

The term "basal body temperature" is defined as the lowest body temperature reached by a healthy person during waking hours. Body temperature varies according to time of day and activity, and for women is affected by cyclical hormonal variations. Therefore, if the two first elements are constant, and the woman is free from infections causing fever, a plotted graph will reflect hormonal activity and so identify the fertile period.

It is best to take body temperatures on waking, at approximately the same time of day, every day. Plotting should be done for six to eight months before users can rely on its accuracy.

Disturbances such as febrile illness, nightmares or disrupted sleep must be indicated on the chart.

Basal body temperature in women normally shows a slight drop at ovulation, followed by a slight rise right afterward which continues to rise until menstrual flow begins.

All that is required for this charting is a BBT thermometer, which is available at drugstores everywhere, along with basal body temperature charts. Temperature may be taken rectally or orally as long as you consistently use the same site. It should always be taken *before* rising. That means before your morning coffee, cigarette or shower.

Many women will register a slight drop in temperature just before or at ovulation. Some however, will note only a 0.4 to 0.8 degree Fahrenheit rise just after ovulation.

Basal body temperature rises only after ovulation. Therefore, if BBT is the only natural family planning method being used, then barrier methods or avoiding intercourse should be practiced until the BBT has remained elevated for at least three days.

The information given in this section cannot be regarded as sufficient instruction for use as contraception; no one method alone is sufficient. Interested couples should see their physicians or attend family planning clinics for thorough instruction.

Remember, any two methods of contraception used together will give you more protection than either will alone.

Further Reading

Anonymous. WHO study finds natural family planning to be "relatively ineffective" even with careful teaching. Fam Plann Perspect 1979; 11:40-41.

Hilgers TW, Prebil AM. The ovulation method—vulvar observations as an index of fertility/infertility. Obstet Gynecol 1979; 53:12-22.

Klaus H, Goebel J, Muraski B, et al. Use-effectiveness and client satisfaction in six centers teaching the billings ovulation method. Contraception 1979; 19:613-628

Wade ME, McCarthy P, Braunstein GD et al. A randomized prospective study of the use-effectiveness of two methods of natural family planning. Am J Obstet Gynecol 1981; 141:368-376.

STERILIZATION

Sterilization as a method of contraception should be regarded as permanent, only to be considered when reproductive capacity is no longer desired. Surgery to reverse vasectomies and tubal ligations, though tried, has had limited success.

Many important questions must be answered before you decide on these methods of contraception. You should discuss these concerns thoroughly with both your partner and your physician.

Do you think you will ever want any more children?

If you should remarry or your children should die, would you want more children?

Do you understand the operative procedures and the changes they cause in your reproductive anatomy?

Are you at all concerned that sterilization may affect sexual gratification or performance?

Only when you, your partner and your physician are satisfied that the above questions have been answered should permanent sterilization be considered. There are no legal limitations as to who can have a vasectomy or tubal ligation—no minimum age, no need to have had children already. It is strictly an arrangement made between an individual or couples and a physician.

Vasectomy

If a couple is considering sterilization, it might be important to know that a vasectomy, male sterilization, is by far the safest procedure. General anesthesia is not required and there are fewer complications than with tubal ligations.

As stated in the chapter *Male Genitalia*, the sperm are formed in the testicles and travel to the outside in two long canals called the vasa deferentia. Interruption of these canals is called a vasectomy (Fig. 6-1). This way sperm, which account for a very small amount of the total ejaculate are prevented from combining with other components at ejaculation. Vasectomy is a relatively simple procedure, usually done under local anesthetic. Small incisions are made in the scrotum, after which the vas deferens on each side is identified, cut and its ends tied. Afterwards there is usually some swelling and discomfort in the scrotal region. Pain is not unlike that after minimal blunt trauma to the scrotum. Some bruising may also appear. Normal activities can be safely and comfortably resumed after two or three days. Following a vasectomy, there will be no change in sexual desire or performance.

Accidental pregnancies after vasectomies are usually caused by failure to follow post-operative instructions. Even though sexual intercourse is allowed after 48 hours, unprotected intercourse should not take place until at least two negative sperm counts are obtained, as sperm may remain in the vasa deferentia for up to ten ejaculations, or eight to ten weeks.

In a very small proportion of men, 1 in 1,000 cases, the vasa deferentia may grow back. For this reason it is advisable, even after two negative sperm counts, to check semen every two to four years.

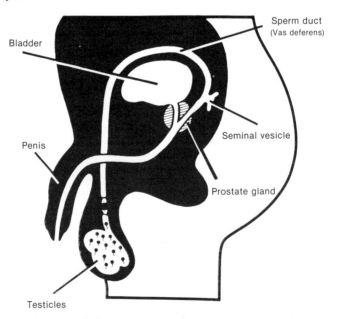

Figure 6-1 Diagrammatic representation of a vasectomy, an interruption of the vasa deferentia (Reproduced with the permission of Wyeth Ltd.)

Surgical procedures aimed at reversing a vasectomy have not met with much success. They are best performed soon after the vasectomy. Only 38 percent of female partners of men who have undergone such a procedure have become pregnant.

Risk Factors

Recently in the press much attention has been focused on two studies that attempt to link vasectomies with the development of arteriosclerosis—hardening of the arteries—leading to heart attacks, strokes or peripheral vascular disease. These studies were done using animal models, i.e., monkeys. Using animal models to predict disease patterns in man can be very misleading. To date, no human studies have found any link between vasectomy and arteriosclerosis. In fact, retrospective studies, which cannot be considered conclusive but only indicative, found that among those men studied who had had vasectomies, there was actually less cardiovascular disease than among the men in the control group, who had not had vasectomies.

Therefore, vasectomy is still considered a safe method of contraception; more conclusive studies will be carried out in the years to come. A man who might hesitate to have a vasectomy because of the possible risk of cardiovascular complications should also consider the greater risks a woman exposes herself to in bearing children, or in undergoing general anesthesia and the more complicated operative procedure known as tubal ligation.

Tubal Ligation

When pregnancies will no longer be desired at any time, many women opt for permanent sterilization (Fig. 6-2). This method is considered 100 percent effective when properly performed.

The basic surgical technique involves ligature, tying or occlusion of the fallopian tubes, so that the ovum and the sperm cannot meet. This can be done via a small incision in the abdomen, called a laparoscopy. The operation can also be done via the vagina and uterine cavity. Some women, after discussion with their physician, elect for tubal ligation during a cesarean section. Many different surgical techniques have been devised over the years. Because increasing numbers of women are

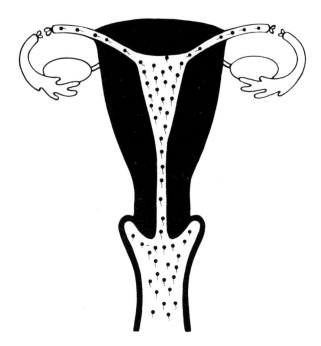

Figure 6–2 Diagrammatic representation of a tubal ligation, the tying or occlusion of the fallopian tubes. (Reproduced with the permission of Wyeth Ltd.)

returning to have sterilization reversed, physicians tend to conserve as much of the tube as possible.

However, tubal ligations should be considered permanent. Some may be surgically reversible, but this cannot be guaranteed.

Finally, because tubal ligation carries greater risk than a vasectomy, couples contemplating permanent sterilization should seriously consider the latter.

Preparing for Tubal Ligation

1. Oral contraceptives should be discontinued one month prior to any elective procedure, including tubal ligation.
2. IUDs removed prior to tubal ligation in order to reduce the risk of post-operative infection.
3. Any possible allergies to anesthetic agents, including family history of malignant hyperthermia, to be discussed with physician prior to surgery.
4. All parties concerned to be well-informed and aware of the permanency of sterilization.

5. Immediately after tubal ligation, possible pelvic pain or discomfort, minor wound pain, shoulder or chest pain due to gas used to insufflate the abdomen during surgery, and possible nausea and light-headedness caused by general anesthesia.
6. Intercourse to be avoided for one week.
7. Wounds in the umbilical area and above the pubis require one week to heal; therefore, heavy lifting during this time to be avoided.
8. Symptoms of complications: high fever, severe or persistent abdominal pain, loss of consciousness, abnormal bleeding, missed periods caused by pregnancy when procedure not properly done.

Further Reading

Price JH. Vasectomy and atherosclerosis. Am Fam Phys 1983: 27:1.

BARRIER CONTRACEPTION

In the early 1970s, when the lay press reported potential health risks from the use of oral contraceptives, there was renewed interest in barrier contraception. Today barrier methods may not represent the most efficient contraceptive mode, but they are gaining in popularity as barriers to sexually transmitted disease. Barrier contraception involves the use of a physical obstruction to prevent sperm from reaching the fertilizable egg. In this group we also include biological and chemical agents that are employed to prevent fertilization.

"Physical" contraception has been documented as far back as 3,000 years ago. Some earlier methods described in the literature include the use of a pessary, a barrier made from dung and honey. This was inserted into the vagina prior to intercourse. In fact, the honey served as a sort of adhesive for sperm. It probably served as a sort of spermicide, as well.

Other agents used in vaginal contraceptives included quinine, rock salt and alum. The earliest, purely mechanical type of barrier for the female was introduced during the crusades, the "girdle of chastity." Various forms of the chastity belt were used to render wives impregnable while soldiers were off at war.

A male counterpart to the chastity girdle was a method used by the Romans called "infibulation." The foreskin was pierced in two places and a ring put through the holes. That way, when the male had an erection, the head of the penis could not clear the ring as the foreskin retracted.

Sea sponges have been used for centuries as a contraceptive method. They were a natural choice, since they were easily acquired from the seabed and could be tailored to fit the vagina. They could be rinsed after each use and used repeatedly. Sponges provided a good barrier, soaking up sperm before they had a chance to reach the cervix.

Douching and vaginal fumigation were popular in the fifteenth century. Different instruments were fabricated to in-

troduce various "medicated" and "anti-human-seed" preparations. Post-coital douches were used by the Egyptians as early
as 1500 B.C. Additives such as garlic, tar, rose petals, pepper,
to name only a few, enhanced the protective effect of douches.

Early precursors of the diaphragm and cervical cap were
used in China and Japan. They consisted of oiled silk paper
placed against the cervix. Later in Europe and Russia, linen cloths
and molded wax wafers were used.

Prototypes of the male condom were made from the bladders of animals, and fashioned to encompass the penis. Ironi-
cally, being ignorant of their contraceptive functions, the Romans
used these early condoms to protect themselves against sexually transmitted diseases

Diaphragm

In 1838, following the discovery of vulcanized rubber, Dr.
Frederich Wilde invented the diaphragm. It gained popularity
in 1882 after a Dr. Hausse wrote a short article, under the name
of Wilhelm P.J. Mensinga, entitled "On Facultative Sterility." It
was a treatise in support of voluntary control of sterility and
included case discussions on the use of the diaphragm. Dr.
Hausse listed the conditions that made voluntary birth control
acceptable:

Permanent. Women suffering from tuberculosis, mental disorders or any other pathological changes as a consequence of
pregnancy or delivery were either unable to bear children or
were advised not to. The diaphragm was recommended to them.

For an undetermined period of time. In the case of diseases
and syphilis, and until recovery occurred, a diaphragm was
recommended to prevent the birth of unhealthy descendants.

For a definite period of time. A diaphagm was to be used
for 18 months by a woman who could not lactate and, therefore, could not nurse her child.

Modern-day contraception would add many more indica-
tions for "facultative sterility."

Use

The diaphragm is the most widely used vaginal barrier (Fig.
7-1). It consists of a shallow rubber cup stabilized by a circum-
scribed rubber-covered steel spring. It offers two-fold protection by acting as a barrier itself and by holding spermicidal gel

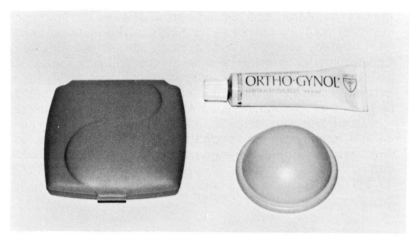

Figure 7–1 Diaphragm and container with spermicidal gel.

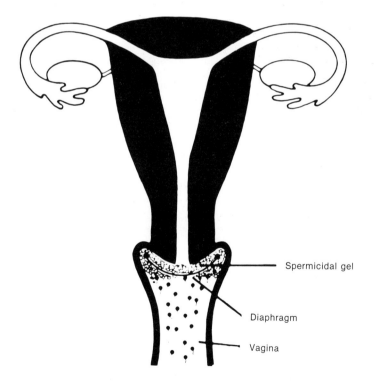

Figure 7–2 Mechanism of action of diaphragm. The diaphragm is placed over the cervical os along with spermicidal gel. (Reproduced with the permission of Wyeth Ltd.)

close to the cervix as a second barrier (Fig. 7-2). Efficacy depends not only on proper positioning but also on an accurate fit. The diaphragm is available in many sizes. It is a very safe, effective method provided it is used correctly. Users should feel comfortable with the device and confident in their ability to insert it and check for proper placement (Fig. 7-3). The diaphragm should be inserted no more than six hours prior to intercourse; it must be kept in place for a minimum of six hours after intercourse. If intercourse is anticipated again within six hours, additional spermicide should be introduced into the vagina without removing the diaphragm.

Pros

1. Ninety-eight percent effective if correctly used; actually 87 percent effective if used with average amount of carefulness.
2. Creates no hormonal change.
3. Causes no serious medical problems.
4. Acts as a barrier to sexually transmitted disease.
5. Barrier methods that prevent STDs may also protect against cervical cancer; studies show cervical cancer acts like a sexually transmitted disease.
6. Temporary, natural and easy to use, convenient and inexpensive.
7. No interference with breastfeeding.

Cons

1. May interfere with spontaneity of sexual activity.
2. May be displaced because of changes in the vaginal wall during orgasm.
3. Ten to 13 percent failure rate considered too high for some.
4. Increases frequency of bladder infections in some women.
5. Not all women can be fitted.

Instructions

Pregnancy that occurs despite the use of the diaphragm usually results from this method not being used consistently. Users have either discarded the device during calculated safe days, or they forgot their diaphragm and/or spermicide while on vacation or away from home for the night.

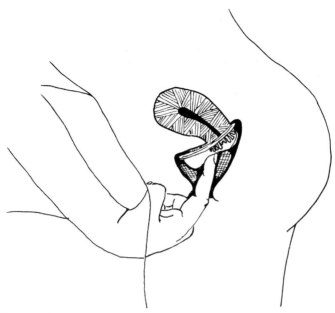

Figure 7–3 Insertion of a diaphragm. Make sure cervix is covered and diaphragm is secure.

It is very important that women practice inserting their diaphragm when being fitted. That way the physician can check to see if it is correctly positioned.

For insertion, about one tablespoon of a spermicidal preparation is applied to the cup of the diaphragm, and some is applied to the rim for lubrication. Opposite sides of the rim are pressed together, so that the diaphragm folds. Using one hand to spread the lips of the vulva and guide the diaphragm, the woman then inserts it so that the cupped portion with the spermicide comes to lie against the cervix. It is then pushed deep into the vagina, the back part of the rim behind the cervix, the front part of the rim behind the pubic bone. The woman should be able to feel the cervix through the soft rubber dome. Occasionally a woman cannot; in this case positioning could be checked by a dependable partner.

After use the diaphragm is easily removed by hooking the front rim with one finger, and then pulling downward and out. It should be washed with plain soap and water, dried with a towel and stored in its case away from heat. It should also be periodically checked for defects such as tears or holes.

If lubricants are used during intercourse, petroleum-based preparations like Vaseline should be avoided, since they will damage the latex of the diaphragm. Many water-soluble lubricants are available at your drug store. If vaginal preparations are prescribed, be sure to check with your physician to be certain they do not contain petroleum.

Problems that may arise and for which a visit to your physician are warranted include:

1. Urinary tract infection; an alternate method may be recommended.
2. Allergy to spermicide; may cause burning and irritation or abnormal vaginal discharge.
3. Inability to properly insert the diaphragm.
4. A missed period; pregnancy must be ruled out before diaphragm use.
5. After pregnancy, surgery of the vagina or weight loss; diaphragm size may change, necessitating refitting.
6. Morning after pill may be necessary if the diaphragm has torn or become dislodged during intercourse.

Cervical Caps

A smaller cup-shaped diaphragm that is placed snugly over the cervix and held in place by suction has recently aroused much interest. It resembles an oversized thimble and blocks the cervix, thus preventing the sperm's access to the vagina. It may be left in place for many days at a time and thus does not interfere with sexual spontaneity. Because of its size, many find it too difficult to handle.

Another reason that it is not so widely used: very few physicians are experienced enough to assure proper sizing and so do not offer the cervical cap to their patients.

Pros

1. Uses less spermicide than the diaphragm.
2. Can be kept in place up to five days.
3. Is inexpensive.
4. Can be put in place long before intercourse.
5. Has no known side effects.

Cons

1.   Develops rubbery odor over time.
2.   General unavailability—manufactured in and imported from Great Britain.
3.   Fitting and instruction for proper use takes several hours.
4.   Occasionally difficult to insert.
5.   Can be dislodged during intercourse, very active sports, coughing spasms or bowel movements.
6.   May cause discomfort and cramping.
7.   Must be tailored to fit each cervix.
8.   Cannot be used by women who are unable to feel their own cervixes.

Vaginal Sponges

Sea sponges have been used for centuries to soak up the semen before it has a chance to come into contact with the cervix. They have the advantage of being relatively clean at the outset and may be used repeatedly. However, there has been no scientific evaluation of their effectiveness. Recently researchers have attempted to produce a collagen sponge that would completely cover the cervix, remain in position, absorb the ejaculate and inactivate the sperm as a result of the collagen's acidity.

The most common complaints to date include discomfort during intercourse and dryness of the vagina.

Modern vaginal sponges are used in clinical studies only and will not be available to the general public until efficacy has been well proven.

Vaginal Chemical Contraception

History tells us that the ancient Egyptians used various substances intravaginally for contraception. Today a wide selection of creams, foams, jellies, suppositories and tablets, known collectively as spermicides, is available (Figs. 7-4, 7-5). These may be used alone but should be used in conjunction with a mechanical-barrier type of contraception. Spermicides have the added advantage of providing a high degree of protection against several venereal diseases.

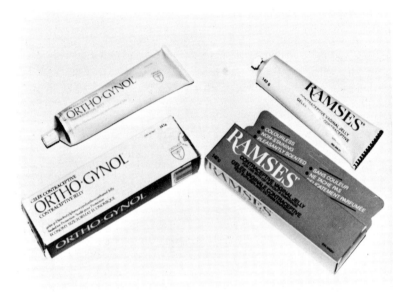

Figure 7–4   Various brands of spermicidal gels.

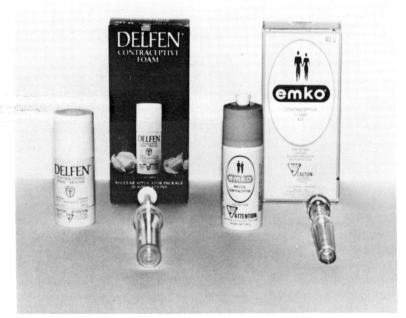

Figure 7–5   Various brands of spermicidal foams.

In 1955, 55 percent of couples practicing contraception used spermicides and/or barrier methods. By 1980, only 18 percent of contracepting couples were using these methods. Many object to the messiness, lack of spontaneity and short duration of action of spermicidal preparations. Yet there are no serious medical complications caused by these products. They do not require a prescription and can be used quite safely by anyone. Allergic or sensitivity reactions in some users are temporary and disappear if the product is discontinued. Often another preparation will not cause the same problems.

As with any other vaginal contraceptive device or preparation, insertion must take place prior to any vaginal penetration by the penis (Fig. 7-6). If foams or jellies are used, application should be deep into the vagina and of sufficient quantity to cover the cervix.

Spermicidal suppositories and tablets recently introduced on the North American market should not be regarded as any more effective than conventional foams. They are, however, less messy. Directions for use of any spermicidal preparation should be strictly adhered to for maximum effectiveness; a new dose should also be used each time you have intercourse. Douching

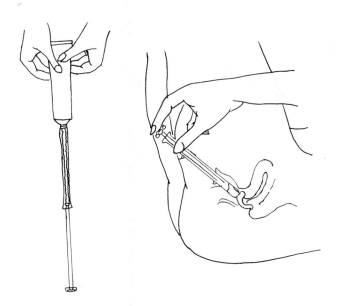

Figure 7–6   Insertion of spermicidal foam into the vagina using an applicator. (Reproduced by permission of Wyeth Ltd.)

should be avoided for at least six to eight hours after the last intercourse since sperm may be forced up through the cervix. If vaginal discharge after intercourse is a problem, a tampon can be used.

Users should be comfortable with their chosen methods. Because these spermicides must be inserted just prior to intercourse, couples must be committed to interrupting foreplay to apply foam, jelly or suppository. This may be awkward in a new relationship and should probably be discussed between sexual partners beforehand in order to avoid embarrassment. Any form of contraception should become a natural positive part of sexual encounters.

Male Barrier Contraception

Condoms were initially designed to protect women against sexually transmitted disease, not as a method of contraception. Ancient Romans used the bladders of animals and fashioned them to encompass the penis.

Condoms were also known as sheaths. Today many would call them "safes," or "sheiks", or prophylactics (Figs. 7-7, 7-8). They are gaining popularity as many women become disenchanted with oral contraceptives or the IUD. Actually, if used properly and in combination with spermicidal preparations, they offer near optimal protection against both pregnancy and sexually transmitted diseases. They are the most widely used form of contraceptive in the world because they are easily acquired, without prescription, and do not require medical supervision to use   Adolescents, who are often too embarrassed to talk about contraception with physicians or counselors, can buy them without hassle. In many major cities and on campuses throughout the world, they can be purchased from vending machines, off the display shelves of drug stores or from super markets. Unfortunately, this cannot be done in all modern centres.

But a popular belief makes condoms less accessible in some societies: the belief that advertising and easy access to condoms arouse sexual curiosity and encourage experimentation by adolescents.

The truth is that unless methods of contraception become more accessible, we will not be able to control the high numbers of unwanted pregnancies among adolescents of this generation. The price for keeping these young people in the dark—unable to contracept freely yet able to sexually interact—is

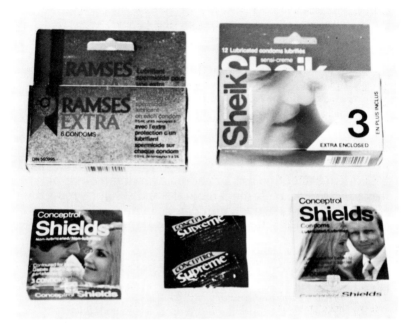

Figure 7-7   Various available condoms.

too high. Mothers, children, and society must pay the price. Studies show that among those adolescents who contracept at the time of first intercourse, the majority use condoms. More would use condoms if they were even more readily available and if instruction prior to use were provided.

Effectiveness

Ideally, when used properly and consistently throughout the menstrual cycle, condoms are 97 percent effective. In practice they are 70 to 90 percent effective, a success rate that can be greatly enhanced by the additional use of spermicidal preparations.

Pros

1. Inexpensive
2. Small, lightweight and disposable
3. Require no medical examination, supervision or follow-up

4. Readily available
5. Provides reliable contraception when properly used, especially when combined with a spermicide
6. No side effects
7. Protects against venereal disease
8. May protect against cervical cancer, since evidence suggests some forms of cervical cancer may be sexually transmitted

Proper Use

For contraception use a condom every time. Several types are available— all must meet federal standards for strength and thickness. Some are even lubricated. In new relationships or in casual sexual encounters, condoms should be used to prevent the potential spread of sexually transmitted disease.

1. Apply condom before vulvar or vaginal contact with the penis.
2. Handle condom carefully, so that it does not tear.
3. Press the air out of the distal tip, leaving about one-half inch at end to hold the ejaculate.

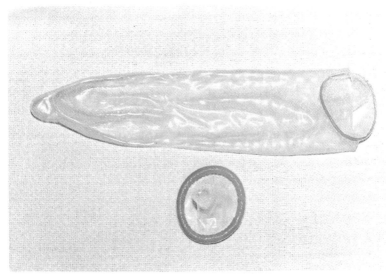

Figure 7–8 Appearance of condom in unrolled and rolled state.

4.   Unroll over as much of the erect penis as possible (Fig. 7-9).
5.   If vagina is dry and condom is not well lubricated, use spermicidal cream or jelly so that friction will not cause tears in the condom or irritate the vagina.
6.   Remove protected penis from the vagina while it is still erect to prevent spillage.
7.   Grip rim of the condom while withdrawing the penis to prevent condom from coming off in the vagina.

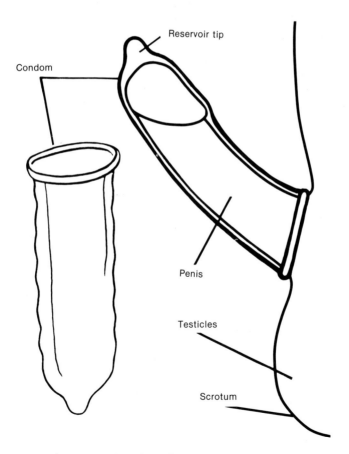

Figure 7–9   Placement of condom allowing about one-half inch at distal tip to hold the ejaculate. (Reproduced with the permission of Wyeth Ltd.)

If the condom is accidentally fitted inside out on the penis, do not reverse it and try again. Throw it away and use another. There is a chance that living sperm were present on the penis and could cause fertilization. If menstruation is delayed, see your physician in the event that you may be pregnant.

A campaign to promote the use of condoms is urgently needed throughout the world to help reduce the growing numbers of people adversely affected by sexually transmitted disease. No sexually active individual is immune to the threat of sterility, sexually transmitted cancers and even death associated with diseases such as condylomata, syphilis, gonorrhea, herpes, chlamydia, hepatitis and AIDS.

Educational and promotional programs should stress the availability, accessibility, acceptability, safety and low cost of condoms.

Condoms are the single most effective barrier against the spread of disease among sexually active individuals. Women should be encouraged to insist that casual sexual partners use condoms, because women in these situations suffer the complications of various sexually transmitted diseases. They may also transmit disease to the unborn or to the newborn. Apart from considering reducing the numbers of their sexual partners, women should use condoms as their greatest protection against infertility and infection.

Further Reading

Alexander JN. Evaluating the safety of vasectomy. Fertil Steril 1982: 37:6.

Cates W. Weisner PJ. Curran JW. Sex and spermicides: preventing unintended pregnancy and infection. J Am Med Assoc 1982: 248:1636—37.

Knes R. The cervical cap. Healthsharing 1982: Fall:17—19.

Smith M. Barwin BN. Vaginal mechanical contraceptive devices. Current review. Can Med Assoc J 1983: 129:699—701.

Tatum HJ. Connell-Tatum EB. Barrier Contraception: a comprehensive overview. Fertil Steril 1981: 36:1—12.

Wright NH. Vessey MP. Kenward B. McPherson K. Doll R. Neoplasia and dysplasia of the cervix uteri and contraception: a possible protective effect of the diaphragm. Br J Cancer 1978; 38:273—279.

INTRAUTERINE DEVICES

An intrauterine device, or (IUD), is a small plastic or stainless-steel object that is placed in the uterine cavity to prevent implantation of the fertilized ovum. In 1977 an estimated 50 to 60 million IUDs were in use throughout the world, mostly in the Republic of China. In the United States, about two million women were using IUDs in 1977.

Over the past century, various sizes, shapes and materials have evolved. The devices currently used are classified as "inert", i.e., non-medicated or "medicated," with copper or progesterone (Fig. 8–1).

These intrauterine devices function as a result of cellular and biochemical changes in the endometrium, the lining of the uterus. They act as foreign bodies, stimulating inflammatory reactions. Such reactions create an environment unfavorable to the implantation of the fertilized ovum. As well, cells mobilized to that area engulf the spermatozoa or the fertilized ovum, destroying them.

The addition of copper increases this inflammatory reaction. Copper itself is also toxic to spermatozoa and so may interfere with conception in other ways.

Similarly, progesterone can be added to the IUD. It is often used in those women who have difficulty tolerating IUDs containing copper. The progesterone causes hormonal changes that disrupt the normal cycle. Menstruations are less painful, and flow is often decreased.

IUDs are recommended for those women who have had a full-term pregnancy and who are in a closed relationship, that is, who have one sexual partner. Often these women are part of a risk group for which oral contraceptives are contra-indicated, or are breast-feeding, or are poorly motivated to use any other method.

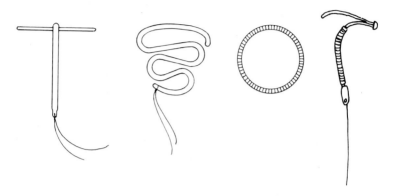

Figure 8–1   Various intrauterine devices:(Reproduced with the permission of Wyeth Ltd.)

Effectiveness

By the end of the first year of use, pregnancy occurs in one out of six per 100 users.

Contraindications

Pregnancy.   The IUD may cause spontaneous abortion, i.e., miscarriage, if implanted in a pregnant woman.

Abnormal uterus.   If the uterus is abnormal in size or shape, the IUD will not fit properly and, therefore, will not exert its desired effect. In such cases, it also may be expelled, or may perforate the uterine wall

History of ectopic pregnancy.   An ectopic pregnancy is one that occurs elsewhere other than in the uterus, usually because of previous fallopian tube damage. IUDs are associated with an increased risk of such pregnancies. The incidence of ectopic pregnancy is 1 percent among the general population and 4 percent among IUD users.

Abnormal bleeding.   The cause of abnormal bleeding should be found and treatment initiated before an IUD is installed.

Presence of infection.   If an IUD is inserted at the time of a vaginal infection, bacterial organisms are more likely to migrate to the uterus from which pelvic infection may spread. Such infections carry a high risk of damage to fallopian tubes and, subsequently, a risk of infertility.

Predisposition to endocarditis. Pelvic inflammatory conditions or manipulation of the cervix for insertion of the IUD may cause infection to be borne by the blood to other sites. Infections of the heart lining, such as endocarditis—infection of the upper lining—are serious and may even be life threatening.

Ingestion of anticoagulants. Bleeding caused by the insertion of the IUD, or subsequent heavy menstrual flow, may become uncontrolled in women on anticoagulants, those agents that prevent normal blood clotting.

Allergy to copper. In the event of an allergy, insertion of a copper IUD may cause reactions that will only subside once the IUD is removed.

Risks of IUD Use

Several recent studies have shown that IUD users run, in general, three times the risk of developing pelvic inflammatory disease (PID), compared to non-users. More significant, however, is the risk of PID in women who have never been pregnant. These IUD users run seven times the risk of non-users. Since pelvic inflammatory disease often leads to fallopian tube damage and, therefore, infertility, the IUD is not recommended for women who have never been pregnant or for those who have multiple sexual partners.

Another risk involved in IUD use is possible perforation of the uterus during insertion, or later, as the uterus contracts on the IUD. Such perforations usually occur if the uterus is small, as in very small women, in women suffering from anorexia nervosa, and in adolescents.

Pros

IUDs have the benefit of being inexpensive. They require only two visits to the physician, one for insertion and one for verification. They need not be replaced for three years if of the inert variety, two years if copper, one year if progesterone. They will not interfere with sexual activity if properly inserted, and their effects are localized to the uterus, allowing for normal cyclical hormonal function.

Insertion of IUD

After discussing this method of contraception with your physician, and if you arrive at a decision to use the IUD, insertion can take place anytime, although it is preferable during menstruation, because the cervix is already dilated to allow for menstrual flow, making insertion easier (Fig. 8-2). Become familiar with the type of IUD your physician chooses for you.

If there exists the possibility of infection from previous sexual encounters, it is wise to request that a culture be done prior to insertion of the IUD to rule out such conditions as gonorrhea.

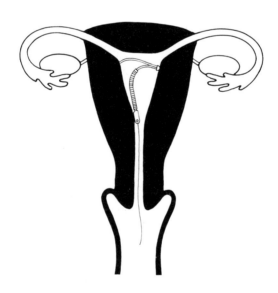

Figure 8–2   Placement of the intrauterine device. (Reproduced with the permission of Wyeth Ltd.)

During insertion the patient may experience sharp cramping pain not unlike that of labor contractions. Some women may "pass out" as part of a reflex caused by manipulation of the cervix and uterus. Afterwards discomfort and abnormal bleeding may continue for several days. Subsequent menstruations may also be prolonged, with heavy flow.

After the first or second cycle a return visit should be arranged to check for proper positioning of the IUD. The physician may choose to do a PAP test at this time. Expulsion rates in the first to third cycles range from 4 to 18 percent. Therefore, it is very important to use a back-up method of contraception for up to three months after insertion.

One way of checking for expulsion of the IUD is to insert one or two fingers into the vagina to check for the string; any changes should be reported to your physician. A missing string may have been drawn up into the cervix or uterus, or the IUD may have been expelled, rendering intercourse unprotected. Out of 1,000 users, in one out of nine cases, the string is lost because the uterus has been perforated and surgical removal of the device will then be necessary.

Occasionally a male partner may complain of discomfort during intercourse if the string is too long or too short or knotted. A revision of the string length may be in order.

Follow-up visits will be required for the following problems:

1. Missed period, to rule out pregnancy
2. Persistent pelvic pain, to rule out infection or perforation of the uterus
3. Abnormal discharge, to rule out infection
4. Missing string, to rule out perforation or expulsion
5. Lengthening of string, to rule out expulsion
6. After possible exposure to sexually transmitted diseases, to avoid PID

Because of the risk of serious infections, IUDs are not recommended for women who have more than one sexual partner or for women whose partners have more than one sexual partner.

Abstinence or No Sex at All

The best way to avoid unwanted pregnancies and sexually transmitted diseases is not to have sexual intercourse at all. Not all physically-sexually mature people wish to be sexually active. Their reasons for abstaining may be personal, moral, cultural or religious.

Even in today's world of sexual freedom and opportunity, there is more and more room for those who wish to put off sexual gratification for the ''right'' moment or the ''right'' person. These people bring to a relationship less chance of having acquired sexually induced infertility, secondary to previous infection of either the female or male reproductive tracts. They are less likely to have suffered the traumas of abortion, of life as a single parent or of having given up a child for adoption.

Abstinence is not a sign of sexual immaturity. Rather, it should be regarded as well-chosen choice, just as sexual activity may be the right choice for someone else.

People who decide to postpone sexual intercourse can still be intimate, expressing feeling through hugging, kissing, hand holding and petting. Such periods may allow a couple time to explore intellectual and emotional boundaries before sexual limits are reached. This way they may test their potential as a couple.

Occasionally one partner might exert pressure on the other to engage in sexual activity for which the other is not prepared. It is important to learn how to say no when appropriate, without causing hard feelings or jeopardizing an otherwise ideal relationship. Ideally, each individual should be able to talk about sexual expectations early, before this situation arises. If you are not prepared or not willing to have intercourse, be firm but kind—if that doesn't work, just be firm! Most any reason used should be acceptable to the other person.

Unreliable Methods of Contraception

Withdrawal. In this case a man withdraws his penis from the vagina before he ejaculates. Withdrawal, or coitus interruptus, is probably the oldest known attempt at birth control. However, it is not reliable, because before a man ejaculates, a drop or two of semen usually escapes from the penis. One drop could contain hundreds of thousands of sperm, and only one spermatozoa is required to fertilize an egg. This method also requires much self-discipline. It has a 15 to 40 percent failure rate.

Douching. This was very popular among Egyptians during the fifteenth century B.C. Several instruments were designed for this purpose, and various additives used to increase effectiveness—garlic, wines, etc. This is not an effective contraceptive method; some studies have found sperm in the uterine cavity within 90 seconds after ejaculation.

Coitus Saxonicus. This involves intercourse until just prior to ejaculation. At this time the female firmly grasps the urethra at the base of the penis, which blocks the forward and outward movement of ejaculation causing it to back up into the bladder. The failure rate is high.

Further Reading

Cardoso R. Intrauterine contraceptive devices. Can Fam Phys 1983; 29:977–79.

Smith M, Barwin BN. Vaginal mechanical contraceptive devices. Current review. Can Med Assoc J 1983; 129:699–701.

Zakin D, Stern WZ, Rosenblatt R. Complete and partial uterine perforation and embedding following insertion of intrauterine devices. (I) Classification, complication, mechanism, incidence, and missing string. Obstet Gynecol Surv 1981; 36:335–351.

SEXUALLY TRANSMITTED DISEASES

A sexually transmitted disease (STD) is an infectious disease that can be transmitted from the host to another person. The contact may be oral-oral, oral-genital, oral-anal, genital-genital, or genital-anal-rectal. Some of these infections can be transmitted via contact other than sexual. As a group STDs have the potential to permanently damage the genital tracts of women and men, leading to infertility. They can affect the unborn and in some cases may cause death.

Since AIDS began to be heavily publicized, STDs in general have become news. Such publicity may cause a panic reaction not at all befitting most conditions. STDs have been with us since recorded time; they will likely remain with us forever. We have survived the scourge of syphilis and gonorrhea; we will survive the threat of AIDS. Many will die because of their exposure to AIDS; more will survive without consequence.

We can minimize the devastation of STDs. The difficulty lies in finding a platform that will unite all groups, bringing about social change that will not undermine the positive aspects of the social evolution we have undergone to date.

The heart of the problem is sex—not the diseases. We could minimize the spread of sexually transmitted disease if only we could all come together and discuss sex and all its implications openly, properly and truthfully instructing subsequent generations.

Unfortunately, today most basic sexual information is still left to parents, the majority of whom are not sufficiently well informed to meet the responsibility they bear. Many young adults—and older adults as well—learn too late about contraception or sexually transmitted disease.

The rise in the incidence of STDs parallels the increase in the number of casual sexual encounters. The group most affected is the 15 to 29 age group. These people come to doctors' offices or hassle-free clinics with very little information about the diseases they have contracted. We must bring information to this group, as few seek to inform themselves. Many are afraid to ask parents, teachers or doctors for fear it will reflect on their character. Still others are oblivious to the dangers of unprotected sex and the ever-present threat of infection.

The psychological effects of these diseases may even overshadow the physical effects. People may not seek medical care out of fear, guilt or embarrassment. And some physicians may not be receptive to their patients' needs, showing disapproval or even hostility towards those seeking information or diagnosis. Such attitudes will further discourage patients from getting the advice and help they need. Fortunately, such physicians are the exception, not the rule.

With changing sexual practices—more casual encounters and diversification of sexual techniques—all social groups are affected by STDs. Adolescents may respond to peer pressure by becoming sexually active. They are usually poorly informed and may only use contraception sporadically, particularly barrier methods, which are known to reduce the probability of acquiring an STD.

Homosexuals represent 10 percent of our society; they are an integral part of any community. Some are married and have children; in fact, 31 percent have sexual contact with women even though they report a preference for homosexual relationships. Homosexual men as a group are at highest risk of acquiring STDs. I must emphasize as a group for many homosexual men do not engage in casual sexual encounters, preferring to be intimate with only one partner. Homosexual women, on the other hand, tend to be more monogamous as a group than their male counterparts. STDs in the female group are much less frequent.

Ninety percent of homosexual men admit to anal-receptive intercourse, as compared to five percent of heterosexual men and women. When anal sex is practiced with large numbers of anonymous partners, a new dimension is added to sexually transmitted disease.

Anilingus—active oral-anal sex also known as "rimming"—has also become more commonly practiced among both heterosexuals and homosexuals. It is easy to see how infectious organisms in stool may pass from one person to another, whether couples are married and monogamous or not. For thousands of years public health officials have been trying to separate human excreta from food supplies and drinking water. Anilingus fosters contamination and is often practiced in casual sexual relationships, resulting in a higher risk of the partners' acquiring infectious agents.

Fecal contamination also occurs when oral-genital sex follows anal-genital sex. Even in oral contacts of genitalia, trace amounts of feces may still be present.

From the above we can begin to understand why the homosexual community in general, because of the number of casual relationships involved and because of sexual practices, is more exposed than most to infectious organisms in general.

Dr. Bell and Weinberg of the Institute of Sex Research in San Francisco studied 5,000 male homosexuals in 1969. Ten percent of the men were involved in "close-coupled" male homosexual relationships. In other words, neither partner sought sexual satisfaction from outsiders. As a risk group, homosexual men committed to each other resemble faithful heterosexual couples—they are at lowest risk.

Open homosexual relationships, characterized by some sexual encounters outside the main relationship, represented 20 percent of those men studied. This intermediate risk group has its parallel in the heterosexual community.

A third and fourth group of homosexual men, known as "functionals" and "dysfunctionals," represented 15 and 13 percent of the studied population, respectively. Functionals are akin to the heterosexual "swinging singles," their lives being organized around more sexual activity, with a greater number of partners. Dsyfunctionals, on the other hand, go from one sexual partner to another, unable to find gratification, yet seeking the security of a close relationship. Both functionals and dysfunctionals engage in more sexual activity and with a greater number of partners than any other group.

But what is important to remember is that the spread of sexually transmitted disease is directly proportional to the number of casual sexual encounters—in any group, be it homosexual or heterosexual. The sexual freedoms acquired in the past two decades have unfortunately served to increase the number of people available for casual sex, and changing sexual practices in all groups have contributed to the spread of various organisms between any two people.

In any community, homosexual or heterosexual, there is a core population, a minority that takes part in anonymous sex and /or group sex. These people are not selective in their choice of partners and do not tend to consider STD risk. They have a higher incidence of STD, and because anonymous sexual contacts cannot be traced, control of disease is virtually impossible. Therefore, even though core populations represent only a small number of heterosexuals and homosexuals, they are responsible for a disproportionately high rate of disease transmission.

If we accept the above, and if we accept that AIDS is one of the sexually transmitted diseases, and if we understand that it is not unique to homosexual men (see chapter 10), then we can appreciate the real threat such a disease could have on the entire community. Studies as early as 1980 showed that 62 percent of homosexual men had decreased their sexual activity by a mean of 24.6 percent. Today even more behavioral change is occurring in that community, reflected in statistics that show a drop in the prevalence in STDs among homosexual men. But for many the change in lifestyle will have come too late. Careful selection of sexual partners and safe sexual practices will save the lives of many more.

We have only to draw this parallel in the heterosexual community: by applying principles of safe sex we can not only decrease the number of unwanted pregnancies, but also the number of STDs.

For years the medical community regarded sexual activity as a matter of personal choice, to be left to one's own judgement. We left the impression that we could always make a patient well, that contact with different individuals held *acceptable* risks. We reinforced that concept in our approach to anonymous sex and to prostitution. Until AIDS sexually transmitted diseases, apart from possible disability from hepatitis, were regarded as inconveniences, unpleasant conditions that could be easily dealt with. This was an innocent oversight. The medical profession felt it had a cure for all STDs. We could deal with all their consequences: we could prescribe antibiotics; we could routinely screen for cervical cancer; we could perform cesarean sections on women who had active genital herpes; we could make test tube babies for those women whose fallopian tubes had been destroyed by pelvic inflammatory disease.

But we *cannot* yet cure AIDS or stop people from dying from this disease.

In reviewing patterns of sexually transmitted disease over the past two decades, you might conclude that things look bad for everyone in society. The more sexually liberated we become, the greater our risk of acquiring sexually transmitted disease. If sexual liberation flourishes among heterosexual groups as it has among the most sexually liberated homosexuals, we will see the same disease patterns emerging.

The time is right for all groups in society—for the medical profession, the educators and the politicians—to join in effecting change.

That change can best be achieved through education. It is difficult for a sexually active person to practice preventative measures if he or she is not sure what ought to be prevented. Young people should be taught about STDs—what they are, how you get them, how they are treated, and most important, how to avoid them altogether. Table 9—1 indicates the prevalence of STDs among patients in STD clinics in the United States.

Table 9-1   The Prevalence of STDs Among Patients in STD Clinics in the United States

Diagnosis	Male	Female
Nongonococcal urethritis	265.3*	-
Gonorrhea	246.7	272.8
Crabs	36.8	24.2
Venereal warts	33.0	36.0
Genital herpes	29.4	18.8
Molluscum contagium	7.7	4.5
Syphilis	7.1	4.0
Trichomoniasis	-	127.9
Nonspecific vaginitis	-	75.0

*Expressed as number of cases per 1,000 visits
Reprinted with permission from the Niaid Study Group, U.S. Department of Health and Human Services, NIH publication No. 81-2213.

It is probably wise for people in uncommitted intimate relationships to restrict their sexual practices to those that carry the least risk of sexually transmitted diseases. They should use condoms or spermicidal preparations to reduce those risks, as well as selecting a contraceptive method that is effective. Only within a closed relationship, when the risk of acquiring a sexually transmitted disease is low, should protective measures be relaxed and less conventional sexual practices be explored.

As women became more liberated and the birth control pill provided them with protection against pregnancy, sexual freedom and expression flourished. Yet women more than men have had to bear the major consequences of sexually transmitted disease. They run the greatest risk of complications, such as sterility and cervical cancer, as well as possibly endangering their newborn.

A new era of caution is in order. Sexually active men and women should apply principles of safe sex.

Each STD now will be described separately. I have attempted to present the material as objectively, accurately and clearly as possible. References will follow every section.

ACQUIRED IMMUNODEFICIENCY SYNDROME

AIDS is the most highly publicized sexually transmitted disease. It is rather unfortunate that the emphasis placed on it has been as a disease mostly of "gays," homosexual men. We know, however, that AIDS afflicts not only promiscuous homosexuals but also promiscuous heterosexuals. It represents a threat to all sexually active individuals who have multiple partners; at least this is what we have observed while studying the homosexual population. Since this is a small closed group, AIDS has been relatively well confined to it. But with increased exposure to the heterosexual population, the disease has and will continue to spread.

In North America, the first cases of AIDS were observed in 1979; on this continent the disease was first recognized as a distinct new syndrome in 1980. Since then, the incidence of AIDS has grown exponentially—5,000 cases in the United States by July of 1984; 10,000 cases by 1985. In Canada, there have been an estimated 650 cases up to the end of 1985.

Because of the virus's long incubation period, changes in sexual behavior today may only be reflected in decreased incidence of AIDS some two or three years down the road.

At first AIDS patients in North America were almost exclusively homosexual. However, groups now at risk include intravenous drug addicts; certain immigrants to North America from countries where the disease is more prevalent, i.e. Haiti and equatorial Africa; hemophiliacs; and newborns or infants of parents in one of the high-risk groups. Understanding the mode of transmission and the origins of AIDS helps us to see why these groups have been singled out.

It is now an accepted fact that AIDS came to us originally from equatorial Africa, or Zaire. History helps clarify how the disease spread. Since diagnostic facilities are not generally available in Zaire, the incidence of AIDS there has been difficult to ascertain. But of 38 cases diagnosed in Belgium in 1983, 31 victims were natives of Zaire. When Zaire gained its independence from Belgium, some say it relied on technical expertise from Haiti—another French-speaking black nation—to train its people. AIDS has a long incubation period, and it is believed that some Haitians, working in Zaire alongside their counterparts, acquired the AIDS virus. When the Haitians completed their training duties, they returned home. This explains why most cases of AIDS among Haitians in Canada and the United States were diagnosed in recent immigrants. Similarly, the immigration of Zairians to Europe explains the high incidence of AIDS among natives of Zaire in Europe.

The Centers for Disease Control (CDC) in Atlanta, Georgia, defines AIDS as "a disease at least moderately predictive of a defect in cell-mediated immunity, occurring in a person with no known cause for diminished resistance to that disease." Such diseases include Kaposi's sarcoma, *Pneumocystis carinii* pneumonia and other serious opportunistic infections.

It is now also generally accepted that the immune defect of AIDS is caused by HTLV-III-LAV, the Human T-Lymphotropic-Virus-Lymphadenopathy Associated Virus, a newly discovered human retrovirus, that is, a human T-cell leukemia virus. The virus was given a name by each of the groups that isolated it: HTLV-III by the American group, under Robert Gallo; and LAV by the French group, under Luc Montaignier of the Pasteur Institute in Paris.

The AIDS virus causes an immune defect in only some of its victims. Many people will contract the AIDS virus without developing the AIDS disease.

Intact T-cell function is a necessary component of the human immune system, which defends our bodies against certain microbes: viruses, mycobacteria, fungi and parasites. In AIDS victims that immunity is impaired and marked by abnormal T-cell function, specifically the destruction of T-helper lymphocytes, known as T4 lymphocytes. Immunosuppression occurs when an individual's ability to fight off infection is compromised. At this point certain malignancies and opportunistic infections strike. These life-threatening infections are caused by organisms that are usually controlled by an intact immune system.

It is not surprising, then, that groups at risk of contacting AIDS include:

1. The sexually promiscuous—since they have increased exposure to infective organisms; to date, homosexuals as a group at greatest risk

2. Intravenous drug users as well as those who get tattooed or have their ears pierced using unsterile equipment
3. Hemophiliacs who use blood products derived from whole blood, prior to July 1985
4. Persons receiving transfusions from AIDS carriers, now screened out through blood testing
5. Children born to AIDS victims, including sperm donors

AIDS is regarded as a fatal disease; most of its victims die within three years. The overall North American ratio is 15:1, male to female.

At the outset the etiology, or cause, of AIDS was a mystery. It was known as the "gay plague." Many theories were examined. Some felt there was a genetic predisposition involved, others that certain recreational drugs were implicated, such as amyl nitrite. Still other researchers believed these individuals' immune systems had been overstimulated by multiple or repeated sexually transmitted infections. The theory is that the immune system becomes overloaded somehow, causing collapse.

The only theory that holds true is the virus theory, which became evident when the occurrence and transmission of AIDS was found to closely resemble that of hepatitis B.

The male homosexual population serves as a good model to examine, hopefully in order to learn about an infectious organism that can spread through any community via sexual contact. We can easily parallel heterosexual behavior to find out what could happen on a national and international scale. Similar behavior will lead to similar consequences—increased promiscuity leads to increased prevalence of STDs, including AIDS. Following safe codes of conduct in sexual matters will reduce the prevalence of STDs, as it already has among the male homosexual community.

In Zaire the male to female ratio of AIDS incidence is 1.1:1, compared to 15:1 in North America. AIDS has the potential of affecting the heterosexual group as well as the homosexual in North America, as it has elsewhere on the globe.

Prior to the AIDS phenomenon, homosexuality itself seemed to be increasing. Homosexuals also appeared to be more sexually active and adventurous and, therefore, were acquiring more STDs.

A discussion of the lifestyles of homosexual men as related to the transmission of disease is limited to only a fraction of the total homosexual population. It excludes lesbians, or female homosexuals, and many who participate in closed relationships.

The core population responsible for a disproportionately high degree of STDs are those 25 percent of homosexuals who have more than 50 different sexual contacts per year. A parallel core population among heterosexuals would be prostitutes, as well some "swinging singles." For a minority in the homosexual and heterosexual populations, sexual promiscuity becomes habit forming and compulsive. It is this compulsive behavior that has become a special problem for the gay community.

In the past, physicians often reinforced the concept that "judicious promiscuity" did not entail unacceptable health risks. Obviously they were wrong. AIDS has made us realize that multiple sexual contacts with different individuals involve significant risk taking. Before the first case of AIDS was diagnosed in 1979, STDs were regarded as a nuisance, yet an acceptable price to pay. Similarly, as other STDs become linked with more serious consequences, such as cancer and infertility, individuals should reassess the situation and make certain adjustments in their sexual practices.

Most homosexual men have altered their habits because of the threat of AIDS. Thousands of men will save their own lives by carefully selecting and decreasing the number of their partners. What is alarming is that heterosexual practices have been changing over the past 15 years, as sexually active adolescents and adults seek to diversify their practices.

We cannot ignore the impact oral-genital contact has on the spread of STDs. The obvious results are best exemplified by the herpes experience. Twenty years ago only 5 percent of Herpes Type I could be found below the belt; it was an oral lesion. Now 40 percent of below-the-belt lesions are Type I, and a proportionate percent of Type II lesions—in the past predominantly below the belt—are now found above the belt.

Studies also show that oral-anal and genital-anal sex are becoming more popular among heterosexuals as well as homosexuals. As many as 25 percent of all North American women have indicated that they have engaged in oral-anal or genital-anal erotic behavior. Since AIDS can be transmitted via blood and sperm, such behavioral changes can only lead to further increases in the prevalence of AIDS among all groups.

Clinical Presentation of AIDS

There are four clinical profiles observed with reference to AIDS.

"Worried Well"

Because of wide media coverage of a disease with so many unknown factors, so many as yet unanswered questions, a group of patients has emerged known as "worried wells." These people are akin to those who suffer from cancer phobia.

The worried well has few sexual partners, is not an intravenous drug user, has no exposure to people with AIDS and has no symptoms. This patient usually does not fit into any group at risk but is extremely concerned that a previous sexual partner may unknowingly have been AIDS positive.

These people are reassured by their physicians and usually offered follow-up examinations and routine screening tests.

Lymphadenopathy Syndrome

This is an unexplained enlargement of the lymph nodes in an individual who is a high risk for AIDS. Such a patient often has some other STD and shows a marginally low helper-T-cell to suppressor-T cell-ratio: T4 to T8. However, this ratio results not from a decrease in T4, but rather an increase in T8. T4 cells have not yet been affected and T8 cells may be elevated in order to mount an immune response against invading organisms.

These patients usually do well. Most do not contract AIDS. We postulate that they overcome initial exposure to the virus, by mounting a sufficient antibody response.

AIDS-related Complex

This condition, ARC, has also come to be known as pre-AIDS, since it has many features of AIDS. The patient has generalized lymph node and spleen enlargement, reduction in T4 cells and reduction in antibodies to fend off HTLV-III, the AIDS virus. The patient may go on to develop full-blown AIDS after a variable period of ill health.

Recent studies suggest that 5 to 20 percent of those with ARC will develop AIDS over a three-year period. Symptoms in this group may include malaise, weight loss, night sweats, diarrhea and extreme fatigue. Patients may even have oral candidiasis. They should be seen frequently by their physicians, informed of their status and urged to seek further medical attention if their condition should change.

AIDS

The AIDS patient will usually describe prodromal symptoms such as enlarged lymph nodes, anorexia, chronic diarrhea, weight loss, fever or fatigue. He or she may have been diagnosed as having ARC in the recent past. It is not known exactly how long incubation lasts before opportunistic infections and related cancers become apparent. Once infection takes hold, the virus may lay dormant, and then later, by some triggering mechanism, destroy its host cell. Many people will have the infection without showing any symptoms, which is the case with many other viral illnesses.

The destruction of the host cell will cause immunosuppression, leaving the patient vulnerable to organisms and certain cancers that are usually easily controlled by the body's defence mechanisms.

Those patients whose first signs of ill health are opportunistic infections seem to have the most severely compromised immune systems. They tend to fare worse than those patients who first exhibit symptoms of Kaposi's sarcoma.

Kaposi's sarcoma occurs in 24 percent of AIDS cases. It is a pigmented purplish cancerous lesion of the skin (Fig. 10-1). In equatorial Africa this condition is endemic, in other words, restricted to that particular region. The sarcoma may be found in other organ systems, especially the digestive tract, as in 50 percent of AIDS cases, or in the lymph nodes. On the skin it appears as a purplish or reddish-blue lesion. It may affect any area of the body.

The CDC in Atlanta has reported a mortality rate for AIDS patients of 21 percent for patients with Kaposi's sarcoma alone; 46 percent for sufferers with *Pneumocystis carinii* pneumonia alone and 59 percent for patients with both KS and PCP. *Pneumocystis carinii* pneumonia accounts for 53 percent of cases of AIDS, while 6 percent of patients have both PCP and KS. Table 10–1 will help clarify the above statistics.

Table 10-1   Mortality Rate for AIDS Patients

	Cases	Deaths	Case-fatality rate, %
KS without PCP	698	148	21
Both KS and PCP	189	112	59
PCP without KS	1,368	628	46
Other opportunistic diseases	423	214	51
Total	2,678	1,102	41

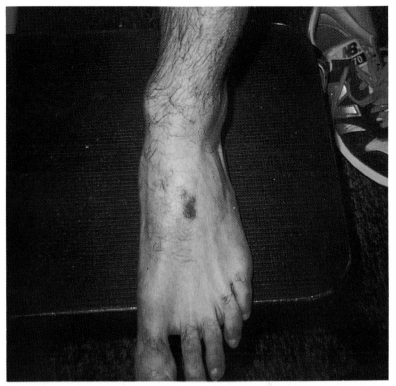

Figure 10-1 Example of Kaposi's sarcoma (KS) on the skin of the foot.

Pneumocystis carinii pneumonia results from an ubiquitous protozoan transmitted by inhalation. A healthy body is able to mount an immune response against this organism; in healthy individuals it will not cause an infection. However, in immune-compromised patients the organism will cause life-threatening pneumonia and symptoms present as a dry non-productive cough and progressive shortness of breath, often associated, as well, with fever and night sweats. Even with treatment, relapses are frequent.

Twenty percent of AIDS patients suffer from other opportunistic infections, such as herpes simplex, oral candidiasis or thrush, which are more extensive and intractable in AIDS sufferers than in healthy individuals.

It is beyond the scope of this book to discuss all possible opportunistic infections, but a list of such organisms would include: *Mycobacterium avium* and intracellulare, *Cryptococcus neoformans*, cytomegalovirus, and multiple enteric pathogens such as *Entamoeba histolytica*, *Giardia lamblia* and *Toxoplasma gondi*.

The fact that AIDS involves many of the body's systems is well documented; for instance, gastrointestinal candidiasis and herpes simplex may also occur, which may then cause a variety of related symptoms.

The central nervous system (CNS) may be affected by cerebral abscesses, resulting in massive headaches, seizures and other neurologic abnormalities. The eyes may be infected as well causing a gradual decrease in visual acuity. AIDS patients typically look chronically ill, thin and weak. They are often lethargic and withdrawn. The median survival time for those proven to have AIDS is only 8 to 12 months; 80 percent of patients die within two years of onset.

Laboratory Diagnosis

At this time there is no definitive, commercially available test to detect the AIDS virus itself, also known as an antigen. The best we can do is to identify those who have been infected by measuring or detecting the presence of antibody to the AIDS virus, HTLV-III. It must be stressed that the presence of antibody does not mean these individuals are not contagious or that they are immune to the disease. If we identify antigens as Ag and antibodies as Ab, a crude table illustrates the possible theoretical outcome of a test to measure both Ab and Ag in a person with a given infection. However, it is not clear once exposure to the AIDS virus and production of antibody occurs whether HTLV-Ag can be destroyed. The time between exposure to AIDS and the detection of antibody in the blood is one to four months. A negative Ab test does not necessarily mean that Ag is not present. Regardless, if the possibility of AIDS contact exists, then Ab testing should be repeated in three to four months. The test model depicted is that used for another virus closely resembling AIDS:

$$Ab/+ \quad Ag/-$$
$$Ab/+ \quad Ag/+$$
$$Ab/- \quad Ag/+$$
$$Ab/- \quad Ag/-$$

Ab Positive, Ag Negative.   This patient, in theory, has rid himself of the virus and is immunized.

Ab Positive, Ag Positive.   This patient's immune system is attempting to mount a defence but Ag is still present and represents a danger of others being infected. The patient could go on to develop AIDS.

Ab Negative, Ag Positive. This patient has contracted the AIDS virus, but the body has not yet gone on to produce antibodies. He-she may go on to develop full-blown AIDS, or at a later date succeed in mounting an immune-defence, hopefully generating enough Ab to destroy all Ag. The patient is a risk to others.

Ab Negative, Ag Negative. This individual shows no signs of having been exposed to the AIDS virus. It is either too early to tell, or the patient is free of Ag. He or she is no danger to others but is the most susceptible to contracting the virus.

Testing for HTLV-III Ab may be recommended for the following groups:

1. Male homosexuals who have been sexually active since 1979
2. Past or present users of intravenous or transcutaneous drugs
3. Hemophiliacs who received blood products or Factor VIII prior to July 1, 1985
4. Persons from areas where the disease is endemic, i.e., Haiti and equatorial Africa
5. Sexual contacts of positive AIDS Ab-tested individuals
6. Children born to parents who are HTLV-III positive
7. Health care workers who may have been accidentally exposed to blood or body fluids of HTLV-III-infected individuals, i.e., pricked with a needle used on an AIDS patient

Screening tests used are enzyme-linked immunoabsorbent assay (ELISA), and Western Blot; immunofluorescent antibody (IFA); or radioimmunoprecipitation assay (RIPA).

Tests results are interpreted in the following manner:

Positive. The presence of Ab to HTLV-III means the individual has been infected with the AIDS virus (commercial testing for antigen, [Ag] is not yet available). Ab-positive individuals should be considered infectious to others. Studies to date have shown the presence of the virus in some HTLV-III Ab-positive individuals for up to five years.

Ab-positive individuals are to take special precautions to prevent further spread of the disease. Positive females should avoid pregnancy.

However, a positive result does not mean you yourself have or will develop AIDS.

Negative. The absence of Ab to HTLV-III may mean that infection via the AIDS virus, HTLV-III, has not occurred or that contact with HTLV-III is so recent that antibodies have not yet formed. It may also mean that infection via HTLV-III has occurred, and the individual's immune system cannot mount enough of a response to produce detectable antibody in the blood.

However, a negative result does not mean that you are not infectious.

It becomes evident that without a test to detect the presence of Ag, not much is gained by informing patients of their Ab status. It is also possible that an individual's Ag-positive status may never be eradicated, because it may be in the nature of the virus to sidestep the body's attempts to destroy it. Ab-positive individuals should consider themselves as being infectious and should take special precautions to avoid spreading the disease.

In different studies among seropositive, Ab positive, homosexual men, followed for 2 to 5 years, more than 50 percent remained asymptomatic, 5 to 19 percent developed full-blown AIDS and 25 percent developed ARC. These statistics are reassuring to some extent, since it seems that AIDS acts much like any other virus—causing clinical disease in only a minority of its victims. Therefore, the majority of exposed individuals probably become immune to the virus.

Yet, until more data are available, and until specific Ag identification can be carried out, all Ab-positive individuals must be considered potentially infectious.

While screening homosexual populations in both large American and Canadian cities, investigators found antibodies to HTLV-III in 50 percent and 15 to 30 percent of gay men respectively. Antibodies have also been isolated in a large number of hemophiliacs and intravenous drug abusers.

Patients thought to be at risk of developing AIDS are usually followed up on a regular basis. They pass a battery of tests to determine a base line state of health. Any irregularities are examined and further testing done. As stated earlier, T lymphocyte, helper-suppressor assays, can be carried out. Abnormal results are suggestive but not diagnostic. Skin tests are done to measure reaction to different common microbial antigens. A lack of expected response is called cutaneous anergy, which is also suggestive but not diagnostic. Other laboratory tests may include biopsy of suspicious cutaneous lesions or lymph nodes. Bronchial washes or lung biopsies may be necessary to isolate *Pneumocystis carinii* pneumonia (PCP).

How Is AIDS Treated?

There is no known treatment for AIDS that will eradicate the infectious organisms or repair the damage the virus has done to the immune system. One can only treat the opportunistic infections and cancers associated with AIDS.

Because Kaposi's sarcoma does not respond to traditional methods of treatment in the area of immunodeficiency, current therapy is largely experimental. Chemotherapy and interferon have been used in the treatment of KS but response is often incomplete and not durable.

Pneumocystis carinii pneumonia can be treated with a combination antibiotic, trimethoprim sulfamethoxazole (TMP-SMZ). It is effective in 50 percent of the cases, but many patients develop severe rashes, in which case another drug, difluomethylornithinel (DFMO), must be used. When TMP-SMZ is well tolerated, repeated PCP infections may be avoided by continuous use of TMP-SMZ.

When any other opportunistic infection is identified, specific treatment can be given. However, the underlying disease remains untreatable.

Almost every major centre is carrying out experimental treatments for AIDS. To date, there is no known cure. Some treatments may prolong life. Some may eventually kill the virus. But damage to the immune system may be irreparable.

Probably the most important aspect of treatment is the care and attention we must pay to the psychological impact of AIDS. The phobia surrounding this disease has isolated this group of patients, not only physically in hospital isolation units, but socially through lost jobs, eviction from apartments and general avoidance by family and friends.

AIDS is not an airborne infection. Healthy individuals are more dangerous to AIDS victims than AIDS victims are to those who are well. Healthy individuals can transmit organisms that are of no consequence to them but that may cause deadly infection in AIDS patients.

You will not catch AIDS except through intimate contact with a victim, through transfusion of AIDS-infected blood or through the use of dirty needles. Casual contact with AIDS victims is safe. Health care workers should refer to their hospital protocol for dealing with AIDS patients. Any other individuals who know an AIDS victim should ask their physician about precautions in order to avoid infecting that patient. Except where sexual partners and children born to infected mothers are concerned, no family members of the more than 12,000 AIDS patients reported to date have contracted the AIDS virus. Some health care workers, including certain physicians, have been reluctant to care for AIDS patients. This is unfortunate. To date, no physician or medical support staff have contracted AIDS in the daily treatment of its victims. This alone should prove that life closely associated with an AIDS victim will not result in contracting the virus or developing the disease. The general population has been very concerned about the spread of AIDS via saliva, tears, urine, etc. Even though presence of the virus in body fluids other than blood and semen has been documented, there is no direct evidence of transmission of HTLV-III virus via these fluids. *You are not at risk of contracting* AIDS *from public pools, restaurants, drinking fountains, etc.*

Homosexual men, who comprise three-quarters of all reported AIDS cases, face special difficulties. These men are often depressed, and because their disease is linked to their sexual activity, they may feel guilty about their homosexuality. Whether they have the disease or not, many have suffered social injustices—being rejected by family, employers and landlords. Fortunately, major cities in the United States and Canada have set up task groups to help AIDS victims, their friends and families.

Prevention

The prevention of AIDS takes four aspects into account:

1. Sexual transmission, including sperm donation
2. Intravenous drug users and their habits
3. Blood transfusions and blood products
4. Transmission to the fetus during pregnancy

Sexual contacts should be chosen carefully. High-risk individuals should practice strict safe sex. They should avoid exchanging bodily fluids, including saliva and semen. The jury is still out on the transmission of the AIDS virus by saliva; it is not likely that concentrations of virus in saliva are high enough to cause infection, but deep, involved kissing should nevertheless be avoided. Those at high risk should also avoid transmission through possible microscopic tears in superficial blood vessels of the rectum or vagina. They should always use condoms for rectal or vaginal coitus, as this may reduce the chance of transmitting the virus.

Those who are aware of their Ab status, who have ARC, or who have full-blown AIDS should not share razors, toothbrushes or any utensils that could be contaminated with blood.

Female contacts of AIDS positive individuals, as well as AIDS positive women, should reconsider having children. AIDS is transmitted to the fetus, so that a child could actually be born with the disease.

Donors to sperm banks should also be selected cautiously; positive donors can infect both the mother and the developing fetus.

Intravenous drug users should be encouraged to use clean needles and never to share paraphernalia.

The likelihood of disease transmission through blood transfusion is slight, but it does occur, and it occurs more often in those areas where donors are paid for their blood. Some IV drug abusers may sell their blood to donating centers in order to finance their habit, and in so doing, transmit the AIDS virus.

Blood donors who are part of high-risk groups should not donate their blood. Laboratory screening tests are now being used to isolate Ab-positive blood from the pool of donors.

There is a fear that certain individuals may purposely donate blood in an effort to find out their Ab status. This could be very dangerous, since Ab testing is not 100 percent sensitive at this time. The Red Cross Society and other agencies must still rely on all high-risk individuals to refrain from donating blood.

Blood products used in the treatment of bleeding disorders have caused AIDS. Their numbers can be reduced by heat treatment of all Factor VIII and Factor IX concentrates. This heat treatment will inactivate the retrovirus. Unfortunately, whole blood and packed red cells cannot be treated in this manner.

Finally, high-risk individuals should not donate organs for transplant. Nor should they undergo tatooing, electrolysis or ear piercing.

One cannot underestimate the impact AIDS could have on our society. It poses a serious threat to us all. It has forced us to rethink our positions on sexuality. More than any other STD it has added impetus to the growing support for sex education in school curriculums.

We owe it to the young to tell them what eroticism and intimacy may involve, so that they may best protect themselves by acting responsibly. If they are not made aware, they may only become aware once their lives have been seriously affected by one or another STD.

Further Reading

Centers for Disease Control updates guidelines for preventing AIDS transmission. Hosp Empl Health 1986; 5:1–4.

Cooper DA, Maclean P, Finlayson R, et al. Acute AIDS retrovirus infection. Definition of a clinical illness associated with seroconversion. Lancet 1985; 1:537–540.

Dotz WI, Bergman B. Kaposi's sarcoma, chronic ulcerative herpes simplex, and acquired immunodeficiency. Arch Dermatol 1983; 119:93–94.

Dunford APJ, Hamilton-Farrell MR, Heath MCD. Acquired immune deficiency syndrome. Br Med J 1984; 288:640.

Durack DT. The acquired immune deficiency syndrome. Adv Intern Med 1984; 30:25–51.

Friedland GH, Saltzman BR, Rogers MF, et al. Lack of transmission of HTLV-III/LAV infection to household contacts of patients with AIDS or AIDS-related complex with oral candidiasis. N Engl J Med 1986; 314:6–7.

Goldsmith MF. HTLV-III testing of donor blood imminent; complex issues remain. J Am Med Assoc 1985; 253:173–181.

Hardy AM, Allen JR, Morgan WM, Curran JW. The incidence rate of acquired immunodeficiency syndrome in selected populations. J Am Med Assoc 1985; 253:215–220.

Harris C, Small CB, Klein RS, et al. Immunodeficiency in female sexual partners of men with the acquired immunodeficiency syndrome. N Engl J Med 1983; 308:1181–1184.

Jaffe HW, Feorino PM, Darrow WW, et al. Persistent infection with human T-lymphotropic virus type III/lymphadenopathy-associated virus in apparently healthy homosexual men. Ann Intern Med 1985; 102:627–628.

Kalish RS, Schlossman SF. The T4 lymphocyte in AIDS. N Engl J Med 1985; 313:112–113.

Kaposi's sarcoma and pneumocystis pneumonia among homosexual men—New York City and California. MMWR 1981; 30:305–308.

Krown SE, Real FX, Cunningham-Rundles S, et al. Preliminary observations on the effect of recombinant leukocyte: A interferon in homosexual men with Kaposi's sarcoma. N Engl J Med 1983; 308:1071–1076.

Leach G, Whitehead A. AIDS and the gay community: the doctor's role in counseling. Br Med J 1985; 290:583.

Levine AS. The epidemic of acquired immune dysfunction in homosexual men and its sequelae—opportunistic infections, Kaposi's sarcoma, and other malignancies: an update and interpretation. Cancer Treat Rep 1982; 66:1391–1395.

Medical News. Acquired immunodeficiency syndrome cause(s) still elusive. J Am Med Assoc 1982; 248:1423–1431.

Mildvan D, Mathur U, Enlow RW, et al. Opportunistic infections and immune defiency in homosexual men. Ann Intern Med 1982; 96(6) Part 1:700–704.

Raphael M, Pouletty P, Cavaille-Coll M, et al. Lymphadenopathy in patients at risk for acquired immunodeficiency syndrome—histopathology and histochemistry. Arch Pathol Lab Med 1985; 109:128–132.

Recommendations of the Centers for Disease Control. Supplement to the January 1986 issue of Hosp Empl Health; recommendations for preventing transmission of infection with human T-lymphotropic virus III/lymphadenopathy-associated virus in the workplace.

Revision of the case definition of acquired immunodeficiency syndrome for national reporting—United States. MMWR 1985; 34:373–374.

Sarngadharan MG, Popovic M, Bruch L, Schupbach J, Gallo RC. Antibodies reactive with human T-lymphotropic retroviruses (HTLV-III) in the serum of patients with AIDS. Science 1984; 224:506–508.

Screening for AIDS? Med Let 1985; 27:29–30.

Vital C, Vital A, Vignoly B, et al. Cytomegalovirus encephalitis in a patient with acquired immunodeficiency syndrome. Arch Pathol Lab Med 1985; 109:105–106.

White GC, Lesesne HR. Hemophilia, hepatitis, and the acquired immunodeficiency syndrome. Ann Intern Med 1983; 98:403–404.

HERPES SIMPLEX VIRUS

Genital herpes now stands as the fifth most common sexually transmitted disease. Over the past decade, the incidence of herpes simplex virus II (HSV-II) has increased markedly, by 20 percent since 1970, depending on the sexual activity within a given population studied.

Herpes simplex II is an incurable and sometimes painful viral infection that may involve a lifetime of recurring attacks. In the United States there are millions of infected people with an estimated 300,000 new cases arising each year. There is a great deal of hysteria about this disease because of the profound way in which it may affect a person's perception of his or her interpersonal relationships. The most serious consequences of genital herpes may be the psychological impact of the diagnosis. Some people are convinced that their lives have been ruined, and they endure the added anguish of feeling like the lepers of biblical times. It has been the press, in great part, that has exaggerated the impact and consequences of this disease.

People with herpes simplex II should be assured that they can lead normal sex lives, without infecting their partners, if they abstain during attacks and do not resume intercourse until 72 hours after the lesions have disappeared.

The disease is a major public health problem because of the symptoms of the acute illness, its tendency to recur, its potentially devastating effect on the newborn, and its association with cervical cancer. The frequency of genital herpes in patients attending STD clinics varies from 1 to 6 percent in males and from 1.5 to 8 percent in females. From patient to patient, there is a wide variation in the clinical manifestations of herpes.

Studies of antibodies to the herpes virus indicate that many people have contracted this disease without any clinical manifestations.

What Is Herpes Genitalis?

Before we can appreciate what herpes genitalis is, we must understand that we are talking about a family—specifically a family of two: herpes simplex I (HSV-I), and herpes simplex II (HSV-II).

Historically, HSV-I has infected the facial area and is known as herpes labialis or, to most, as cold sores. Recurrent herpes simplex labialis affects 20 to 45 percent of the North American population. Approximately one-quarter of those afflicted have three or more recurrences per year. HSV-II infects mainly the genital area and has come to be known as herpes genitalis. However, either HSV-I or HSV-II can occupy both the area above and below the belt, and clinically it may be very difficult to distinguish one from the other.

The herpes viruses belong to the group herpes Viradea, which contains HSV-I and HSV-II; varicella-zoster, chicken-pox; herpes zoster, shingles virus; cytomegalovirus; and Epstein-Barr, mononucleosis virus.

In lower socioeconomic groups, HSV-I infections, as documented by the presence in the blood of antibody to the virus, occur in children before the age of five. Prevalence rates of specific antibody to HSV-II—depending on socioeconomic status, past sexual activity and locale—range from 10 to 77 percent (Romanowski). With changing sexual practices, i.e., oral genital, herpes labialis, HSV-I, may account for 20 to 50 percent of genital lesions.

So genital herpes is a viral infection of the genital area by either herpes simplex I or herpes simplex II. The virus enters the cell, causes a blistering infection and then is dormant until reactivated. Once HSV has invaded the host, it can make its way up the nerve, innervating a given area, then hide there and remain latent long after any signs of active infection have disappeared. Later the virus travels back down the nerves to the affected area to cause a recurrent herpes infection.

How Does One Get Genital Herpes?

Herpes simplex viruses I and II are normally transmitted through direct intimate contact with infected areas. This contact is usually sexual—oral-oral, genital-genital, genital-oral, genital-rectal or oral-rectal. You can also catch herpes simplex by touching an active lesion or fluid-filled blister, and then soon after, touching a part of your body or somebody else's. Herpes infections of the eyes can also be caused by autoinoculation, the act of infecting oneself. For example, never use saliva as a wetting solution for contact lenses. If the infectious fluid has time to dry, it becomes non-infectious; the virus is killed. Therefore, it is not likely that you will catch herpes from toilet seats or chairs.

Since heavy loads of virus may be shed from open lesions, infection may be transmitted to susceptible persons via fingers or hands or close body contact, e.g., mothers to children. However, as genital herpes lesions are usually covered by clothing, they are less of a risk to family and friends than herpes on the lip.

Persons with prior HSV-I infections can also acquire HSV-II, and vice versa. These secondary infections, known as non-primary first episodes, have a slightly shorter course than a true primary infection would.

Recently articles have appeared stating that HSV can survive on toilet seats for up to 90 minutes. This is interesting theoretically only because transmission by this means has never been documented. Also reported has been the fact that 0.65 to 15 percent of adults may be excreting HSV-I or II at any given time, depending on the population being studied. In women, this may take the form of asymptomatic herpetic lesions and transient shedding of HSV from the cervix or vulva without obvious lesions. It is not yet clear what role asymptomatic viral shedding might play in the contracting of either virus. In summary:

1. HSV-I or II may indiscriminately infect the areas above and below the belt.
2. Autoinoculation is not uncommon and must be considered a risk.
3. Transmission may occur via oral-oral, genital-genital, genital-oral, genital-rectal or oral-anal contacts.
4. Transmission may be non-sexual.

What Are the Symptoms?

The first, or primary, infection of herpes simplex I or II usually becomes evident within seven days after sexual intercourse or oral-genital contact; it will last up to three weeks. Lesions appear as small blisters and are often itchy. They look like Garden-variety cold sores. The blister will often break and then fade to a gray-based ulcer.

These lesions most often occur singly or in clusters on the perineum, vulva, vagina, and/or cervix, penis, thighs or buttocks (Figs. 11-1 to 11-3). They are usually painful, but since the cervix and the upper two-thirds of the vagina have practically no sensitivity, lesions in this area may be painless. The lesions usually form scabs and heal in three to four weeks.

Primary genital herpes may often include systemic symptoms such as general malaise, muscle aches, low-grade fever, headaches, and swollen lymph glands. Recurrent herpes genitalis infections are accompanied by fewer lesions that last about 10 days. At least 60 percent of patients with primary genital Type

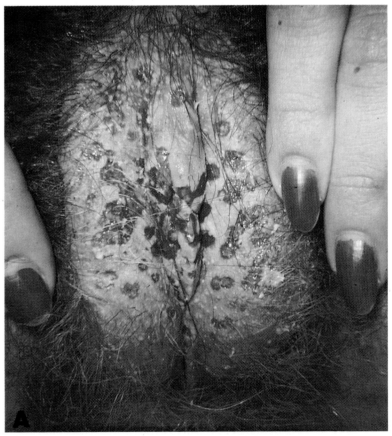

Figure 11-1 *A,* Herpes vulva superficial hemorrhagic ulcerations. (Reproduced with permission of The American Academy of Dermatology.)

II herpes develop recurrent genital infection within six months following the primary episode; 75 percent of patients develop recurrent infection within a year. As many as 30 percent of patients who suffer a first attack never experience further attacks.

Recurrence of HSV infections is explained by the term latency. At present, there is little evidence of continual production of infectious particles between episodes of acute infection, i.e., during latency.

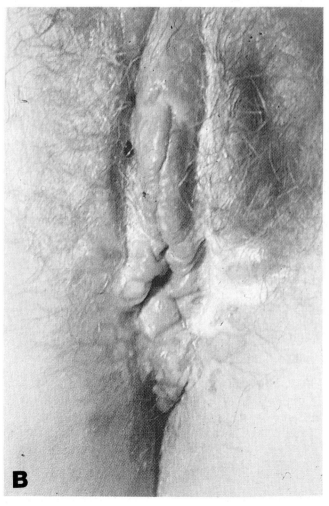

Figure 11-1 *B.* Herpes vulva–healing ulcer craters. (Reproduced with permission of The American Academy of Dermatology.)

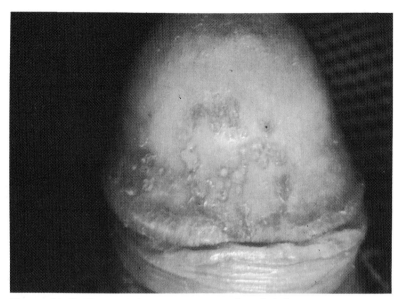

Figure 11-2 Herpes—glans penis. (Reproduced with permission of The American Academy of Dermatology.)

There are two theories about latency that help to explain the recurrence of HSV infections. The "static theory" is that the quiescent, latent virus is somehow "switched on" to initiate an active infection. Viral particles are then transported down the nerve root to the skin, where they multiply and a lesion results. The "dynamic theory" holds that local host immune mechanisms continually suppress viral replication, a process known as autoreproduction. Lesions occur when something happens to overwhelm this local immune response. It is not known what really triggers recurrences of genital herpes. However, of those patients studied who have identified precipitating factors, most cited emotional stress; others stated that recurrences were related to menstruation, sunlight, fever or local trauma, intercourse being an example of the latter.

A complicated symbiosis between a virus and its host allows viruses to live with us for decades. We carry on with our lives and they periodically reactivate.

Recurrences vary in frequency, from more than one attack per month, 5 to 25 percent incidence, to more than one attack every six months, or 10 to 65 percent. As time goes on, there is usually a greater span between recurrences; symptoms dimin-

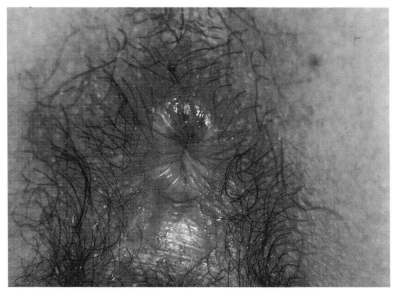

Figure 11–3 Herpes genitalis—anal lesion. (Reproduced with permission of The American Academy of Dermatology.)

ish, and healing time is reduced. One-third of men with recurrent disease never experience pain. Virus is shed for only 4 to 5 days, and the infection is over in 9 to 10 days.

For the majority of women studied, the recurrence of genital herpes infection was minimal in its effects. Pain lasted an average of four days and was described as mild. The average healing time was eight days. Sixteen percent of women with recurrences shed virus from lesions after 6 days and, therefore, continued to be infectious. Cervical shedding has been observed in 33 percent of patients during recurrence and in four percent of patients between recurrences. Although the risk of transmitting HSV through sexual intercourse during asymptomatic periods is not known, low levels of virus found in the absence of lesions suggest that the risk is small.

Unlike the primary infection, recurrent infection is often marked by a prodrome, a symptom of impending infection. People may experience an itching or tingling sensation for a few hours to a day before the appearance of active infection. They may complain of pain extending to the buttocks or even the knee, described as a neuralgia. These symptoms subside with the appearance of blisters.

Neuralgia, then, or the prodrome, is an important event, because it tells you that you may be having a recurrence and that, in order to decrease the risk of transmitting infection to others, you should not engage in sexual activity. Intimate contact should not resume until 72 hours after lesions have disappeared.

Diagnosis

If you experience any of the symptoms described, you should consult your physician for diagnosis and instructions. A diagnosis may be clinical; an experienced physician may not require laboratory confirmation if the history and physical examination leave little doubt in his mind. A negative laboratory test in light of previous examination by the physician may, in fact, be a false-negative.

However, a physician may use any one of three tests—immunofluorescence, Papanicolaou and crystal violet—for diagnosis. The most definitive test, though, is isolation of the virus in tissue culture.

Treatment

While many treatments for genital herpes have been written up in the scientific and lay press, so far no procedure has eliminated latent viral infection. Symptomatic relief through analgesics and local care are all that can be offered. If you are infected, keep the area dry and be reassured that the condition has built-in limits. Saline soaks, salt solution, may be helpful.

Some treatment modalities are worth mentioning and so will be briefly discussed.

Acyclovir (Zovirax) is a commercially available drug that appears to shorten the course of the disease and relieve symptoms. But it does not bring about a cure. It is most effective in a first attack and may reduce the period over which viral shedding from herpetic lesions occurs, thus shortening the patient's infectious period.

For maximum benefit, acyclovir should be used as soon as possible after the onset of an infection, i.e., within eight hours after the onset of lesions. Primary infections benefit the most from the drug. In the event of recurrent infection, acyclovir as a topical preparation offers only a modest benefit. Acyclovir is now being marketed in the United States in an oral form, as a preventive treatment for recurrent herpes. It has also been successfully used intravenously by patients hospitalized with severe HSV infection.

Beware! There are many ineffective therapies being offered to people. A review is needed here, since many people will try these out of desperation.

Vaccines. There are no approved vaccines in the United States and Canada.

ANTIVIRAL AGENTS

Acyclovir. As previously discussed, this antiviral agent does have limited value in controlling infection, but it will not effect a cure.

Vidarabine. Used in the treatment of eye infection and encephalitis this agent is useful, but is not effective in the treatment of genital herpes.

Idoxuridine (Herplex-D, Stoxil). Idoxuridine has been shown by many studies to be useful only for treating eye infection; therefore, it is not useful for genital oral herpes infection.

Ether, vitamin therapy, lactobacillus, zinc, lysine, dye-light therapy, silversulfadiazine, nonoxynol—none of these preparations is effective in the treatment of genital herpes. Some may even be harmful if not properly used.

Dimethyl Sulfoxide (DMSO-Rimso-50). This antiviral agent is a liquid solvent, that when used alone, has no proven effectiveness. However, when used in combination with topical, antiviral compounds, it may increase the penetration of the compounds into the skin, thus increasing its effectiveness.

Providone-Iodine (Proviodine, Betidene). Providone-Iodine preparations are only good as antiseptic and drying agents, but they do not help heal HSV lesions more rapidly.

2 Deoxy-D-Glucose. This is a chemical agent currently being tested for treating HSV infections. Its effects are not yet known.

Associated Health Risks

The "hysteria" associated with herpes derives its force from the fact that HSV infections are a never ending nuisance. In an era of sexual freedom and promiscuity, people are still traumatized by the labels "venereal" or "sexually transmitted diseases." The fact that one must live with the label "herpes" for a lifetime appears to some as an unfair reflection on them and their behavior. The truth is that it is fairly difficult to escape the reality of genital herpes infections. Up to 50 percent of the North American population has been proven to be carrying viruses, either HSV-I or II, facial or genital. As sexual habits change more and more, viruses that were facial are being transmitted to genital areas, while more genital viruses are being transmitted to facial areas.

A great deal of counseling is required for those people who have discovered they have herpes, and much more remains to be done to make our society more accepting of those who know they are HSV carriers. We must remember that a great many people are carriers who are unaware of their status; they may pose a great risk to others.

Herpes is a nuisance infection for the majority of people. With proper follow-up and care, major complications can be avoided.

Herpes Encephalitis

This infection of the brain is a very rare complication resulting from direct viral invasion. Untreated, it has a mortality of 70 to 80 percent.

Herpes Meningitis

More common than encephalitis, this infection of the brain covering may occur in four to eight percent of cases. Patients suffer with nuchal, neck, rigidity; fever; photophobia, abnormal sensitivity to light; vomiting; and severe headaches. The condition is benign. Patients are usually hospitalized, and the disease, with proper treatment, resolves itself.

Herpes in Pregnancy

There is a risk of passing HSV from active lesions to newborns as they move through the birth canal. The event is rare, accounting for 700 cases annually in the United States and 40 annually in Canada. When infection of the newborn does occur, 40 to 60 percent suffer severe or fatal disease. Because of the threat of encephalitis, cesarean section is recommended as a mode of delivery for patients with active infection.

It is possible to minimize the risk by informing your physician of your health status. That way, he will follow the pregnancy more closely. Only women who are shedding virus at the time of delivery transmit virus to their infants. Therefore, by proper screening, culture and PAP smear, measures can be taken to prevent transmission.

Herpes recurrences during early pregnancy probably have no real effect on the outcome of the pregnancy. The developing fetus seems to be well protected in its environment, i.e., enclosed in fetal membranes.

It should be emphasized that having genital herpes does not necessarily make cesarean section inevitable. Only those women shedding HSV at term will require it.

Breast feeding is allowed for women who have herpes, provided that there are no herpetic lesions in the area and that exposed, active lesions elsewhere are well covered. This includes facial lesions. Breast feeding mothers should be taught proper hand-washing techniques and protective measures.

Women with HSV are no danger to other women and may remain on maternity wards without fear of contamination of others.

Complications in newborns exposed to HSV are greatest in the premature group and may also occur anytime during the first month of life. Newborns who survive HSV infection without severe complications develop recurrent infections, much like adults.

A pregnant woman with genital herpes is two to three times more likely than a non-infected woman to experience a spontaneous abortion, i.e., miscarriage, or to deliver a premature infant.

Herpes Link to Cervical Cancer

A link to cervical cancer, though unproven, is suspected. For this reason, regular PAP smears are advised for those women with the virus. The risk seems to be low and is affected by the age of the women at the onset of intercourse and by the number of sexual partners. All women who have sexually transmitted disease are at increased risk of cervical abnormalities.

Kessler, in a review of evidence to date, lists both direct and indirect evidence implicating genital herpes virus, HSV-II, in cervical cancer.

Indirect Evidence

1. HSV-II has been proven to be a venereally transmitted virus.
2. Cervical cancer "behaves" as a venereal disease.
3. Its occurrence is correlated to that of penile cancer in males.
4. It has often been found in patients who have a variety of other venereal diseases.
5. Our prospective study of the male role in cervical cancer suggests that if a woman marries a man who was once married to or who will later marry a woman who developed cervical cancer, the man's present wife runs a two to three times greater risk of developing cervical cancer herself.

Direct Evidence

1. HSV-II has been isolated in the genitourinary tract, the prostate, vasa deferentia and urethra of 15 percent of male urology clinic patients.
2. Followed prospectively, biopsied cervices showing evidence of active herpetic infection developed cervical cancer of atypia in nearly one-quarter of the cases.
3. There is significantly increased prevalence of neutralizing antibodies against HSV-II among women with cervical cancer.
4. Exfoliated cervical cancer cells reveal through the immunoflourescence test, HSV-II antigens.
5. Cervical cancer biopsy tissue can be induced to release HSV-II virions and/or infectious virus.
6. HSV-II viral DNA and messenger RNA have been detected in cervical tumor tissue.
7. HSV-II antigens are associated with active growth of cervical tumors. Kessler, 1979.

Whatever the pathogenic factors in human cervical cancer, early detection through screening remains the best method for prevention of mortality and morbidity.

And the data should be reviewed cautiously. Even though many fingers point to HSV-II as a predisposing factor in the development of cervical cancer, these studies are not conclusive, since both cervical cancer and HSV infections have the same predisposing factors. Both occur in women who are sexually active at an early age. Both occur in women who have multiple partners. Both occur in women who have frequent intercourse.

To be on the safe side, women who have had herpes infection should have PAP smears, checks for cervical cancer, at least once a year. Early detection can cure cervical cancer.

What Do You Do if You Have Genital Herpes?

It is difficult for sexually active individuals to ensure that they do not acquire genital herpes, given the fact that 300,000 new cases are diagnosed in the United States each year, and that up to 50 percent of the population has developed antibodies to HSV-I or II.

One should choose sexual partners carefully—inquire about possible past history of HSV infection, understand the disease. If you are not sure about a new partner's "sexual pedigree," you should insist on the use of a condom to guard against sexually transmitted disease. A person with active genital herpes should avoid sex but need not avoid other forms of intimacy.

A positive approach to HSV is very important in order to avoid or minimize adverse psychological reactions in those with the infection. Hopefully, physicians will be able to reassure those affected by taking time to discuss completely the implications of the disease.

How To Inform Your Sexual Partner

(from the publication "Coping with Herpes," by R.E.A.C.H.)

Where?   In an environment where you are both comfortable and relaxed. An environment that allows both of you to freely communicate your thoughts and feelings.

When?   When contact with the infected area is a genuine possibility, and when you can both be alone, uninterrupted and unhurried.

How?   Openly and honestly. You need not blurt out, "I have herpes," but a question such as, "Do you know what herpes genitalis is?" may serve as a starting point. You might present both the pertinent positive and negative facts without emphasizing either, e.g., "I can have children, but a cesarean birth may be recommended by my doctor." Try to be fair and balanced.

Neutral, factual and nonjudgmental expressions—both positive and negative—are most appropriate. For example:

Extreme: "I have an incurable disease."
Neutral: "Although there is no cure for herpes, with proper care and management, it is no great threat to you or me."
Extreme: "I am contaminated."
Neutral: "When I have lesions, I can transmit the disease through intercourse or oral sex, but when the lesions are not there, the possibility is minimal."

If you are unaware of some aspect, say so; inaccurate information can create false hope or unnecessary fear. Avoid self-deprecating remarks, especially labels. For example, "I have a disgusting disease that has turned me into a social leper," versus "I have a virus that acts up sporadically." Refuse to be defensive, self-pitying, demanding, etc. Share pamphlets, fact sheets and any other information on herpes with your potential partner and encourage him or her to ask questions and express feelings.

What to expect.   The person being confronted may have many questions and may not be able to make an immediate decision. The potential partner may also have herpes.

Once everything has been said, someone with herpes may still be rejected as a sexual partner; however, it is important to realize that not everyone has the same response. If the person with herpes adopts a positive attitude regarding him- or herself and the illness—that herpes is not a terrible phenomenon and that he or she is still a complete person—others will like-ly assume the same attitude and treat the person accordingly. It is sometimes difficult to be objective when the issue is so personal; therefore, support and encouragement may be needed to promote a positive attitude.

Further Reading

Aurelian L. Possible role of herpesvirus hominis, type 2, in human cervical cancer. Fed Proc 1972; 31:1651–1659.

Brown ST, Jaffe HW, Zaidi A, et al. Sensitivity and specificity of diagnostic tests for genital infection with herpesvirus hominis. Sex Transm Dis 1979; 6:10–13.

Chang T, Fiumara NJ, Weinstein L. Genital herpes: some clinical and laboratory observation. J Am Med Assoc 1974; 229:544–545.

Committee of Fetus and Newborn, Committee on Infectious Diseases. Perinatal herpes simplex virus infections. Pediatrics 1980; 66:147–149.

Corey L. Genital herpes. In: Holmes KK, Mardh P, Sparling PF, Wiesner PJ, eds. sexually transmitted diseases. New York: McGraw-Hill, 1984; 449.

Corey L. The diagnosis and treatment of genital herpes. J Am Med Assoc 1982; 248:1041–1049.

Guinan ME, MacCalman J, Kern ER, et al. The course of untreated recurrent genital herpes simplex infection in 27 women. N Engl J Med 1981; 304:759–763.

IC officers must recognize herpes to control spread in hospitals. Hosp Infect Control 1981; August:103–105.

Kawana T, Kawagoe K, Takizawa K, et al. Clinical and virologic studies on female genital herpes. Obstet Gynecol 1982; 60:456–461.

Kessler II. On the etiology and prevention of cervical cancer - a status report. Obstet Gynecol Surv 1979; 34:790–794.

Kibrick S. Herpes simplex infection at term: what to do with mother, newborn, and nursery personnel. J Am Med Assoc 1980; 243:157–160.

Nahmias AJ, Roizman B. Infection with herpes-simplex viruses 1 and 2 (first of three parts). N Engl J Med 1973; 289:667–674.

Nahmias AJ, Roizman B. Infection with herpes-simplex viruses 1 and 2 (second of three parts). N Engl J Med 1973; 289:719–725.

Nahmias AJ, Naib ZM, Josey WE. Epidemiological studies relating genital herpetic infection to cervical carcinoma. Cancer Res 1974; 34:1111–1117.

Romanowski B, Sutherland R. Epidemiology and control of sexually transmitted diseases. Med N Am, Infect 2 1983; 6:494–498.

Whitley RJ, Nahmias AJ, Visintine AM, Fleming CL, Alford CA. The natural history of herpes simplex virus infection of mother and newborn. Pediatrics 1980; 66:489–494.

Yonekura ML. Doctor warns against overreaction to genital herpes. Occup Health Nurs 1982; August:40–41.

CHLAMYDIAL INFECTIONS

What Is Chlamydia?

Chlamydial infections of the cervix, urethra and rectum are the most prevalent sexually transmitted diseases, STDs, in Canada and the United States, afflicting a total of three million per year. They frequently lead to serious complications, including pelvic inflammatory disease (PID); epididimytis; and proctitis. *Chlamydia* is also responsible for the disease trachoma, which remains one of the world's leading causes of preventable blindness.

Chlamydia trachomatis is an obligate, intracellular parasite. In the past, and even today to some extent, it has been a very difficult organism to isolate, thereby making it difficult to diagnose infected individuals.

In men, *Chlamydia* accounts for 40 percent of urethritis cases not related to gonorrhea.

Infants may acquire this infection while passing through the birth canal, later developing inclusion conjunctivitis, eye infections, which affects 50 percent of infants whose mothers have the infection, and pneumonia, which affects 20 percent. In those women not using barrier methods of contraception, the risk of chlamydial infection increases with the number of sexual partners. Multiple partners explains the higher prevalence of *Chlamydia*, up to 20 percent, among women studied at STD clinics and among women receiving prenatal care at public hospitals in the United States in 1980.

What Are the Symptoms of Chlamydial Infections?

Most women with chlamydial infections are asymptomatic, i.e., they have no symptoms. Some may experience painful urination, abdominal pain, abnormal vaginal discharge and deep pelvic pain during intercourse. But please note that these symptoms are very nonspecific and are reported with similar frequency by noninfected women.

Men may also be asymptomatic, i.e., 25 percent have no symptoms, or may complain of burning on urination or a clear to milky urethral discharge. Chlamydial infection accounts for 40 percent of nongonococcal urethritis and 60 percent of postgonococcal urethritis in those who were once infected with gonorrhea but continue to have symptoms of urethritis.

For those women and men practicing anal intercourse, chlamydial infections are usually asymptomatic, rectal infections. These people may complain at times of rectal pain or changes in bowel habits.

How Is Chlamydia Diagnosed?

Although classified as a bacterium because of its cell wall chemistry, *Chlamydia trachomatis* is an obligate, intracellular parasite and so requires a cell culture host system for its isolation. These culture requirements are not widely available, so that diagnosis and treatment are usually based solely on the presence of clinical symptoms. However, this method deals with symptomatic patients only and does nothing to find the 5 to 20 percent of men and women who make up an ever-expanding reservoir of those who risk the most serious complications of chlamydial infection.

Chlamydia trachomatis has been isolated in approximately 5 percent of female college students in the United States. Antibody to *Chlamydia trachomatis* was found in vaginal secretions in up to 12 percent of the women who requested routine medical examination.

To date, there is no feasible way of detecting these carriers, but screening high-risk individuals and symptomatic patients will help control this infection. A physician is often able to make a presumptive diagnosis after examining the patient and taking an appropriate medical history.

Blood tests, microbiological isolation and cytological techniques often have not been available , or available only in some areas. Specific changes in PAP smears are felt to correlate well with chlamydial infections; PAP smears are thus often useful in diagnosis.

A direct test on clinical specimens—vaginal-endocervical and urethral—using fluorescein-labelled monoclonal antibodies to *Chlamydia trachomatis*, is now available. The test is called Microtrak. If properly done, it has an overall sensitivity rate of about 95 percent and a specificity of about 99 percent. Microtrak is a rapid alternative method for the detection of *Chlamydia trachomatis*. It is commercially available and easy to use. As health protection laws are updated, *Chlamydia trachomatis* will become a reportable disease along with gonorrhea, syphilis and other communicable diseases. This way, the medical profession will be able to more accurately define the incidence of chlamydial infection and treat contacts, in an attempt to reduce the incidence through identification of asymtomatic carriers.

How Is Chlamydia Trachomatis Treated?

Urethral, cervical and rectal infections caused by the disease are treated with tetracycline, erythromycin or their derivatives. Rectal, epididymal or testicular infections are treated for a longer period of time. Pelvic inflammatory disease is usually treated on an inpatient basis, in the hospital.

What Are the Possible Complications of Chlamydia Trachomatis?

As with most STDs, the possible complications overshadow those that actually occur. Once again, women suffer the most, since possible consequences include both upward spread of the disease to the pelvic area and infection of the newborn.

Pelvic Inflammatory Disease

Infection of the uterus, endometritis, or the fallopian tubes, salpingitis, are the most common complications of *Chlamydia trachomatis* infection. Up to 60 percent of those with PID may have *Chlamydia trachomatis*.

While oral contraceptives may offer some protection against gonococcal PID, gonorrhea, it is not yet certain—it may even be unlikely—that the pill provides a similar protection against chlamydial PID.

Treatment of this disease usually requires hospitalization. For more information, refer to the chapter *Pelvic Inflammatory Disease.*

Infertility

As noted above, chlamydial infection may spread to the fallopian tubes, causing scarring or blockage, thus preventing the normal passage of egg and/or sperm for fertilization. Infertility is, therefore, often the first indication that a chlamydial infection has occurred.

Studies confirm that past chlamydial salpingitis is associated with the development of peripheral fallopian tube obstruction, with resultant infertility.

Postabortal Pelvic Infection

One-fifth of PID cases after miscarriage or abortion are associated with *Chlamydia trachomatis.*

Infant Disease

It is well known that *Chlamydia* can be transmitted to the newborn as the infant traverses the birth canal. The infection causes infant pneumonitis, pneumonia, and conjunctivitis, and is suspected of causing otitis media and gastroenteritis. Very few of such illnesses require hospitalization.

Prevention

The rules that apply to other STDs apply to *Chlamydia trachomatis,* as well. Means of avoiding the disease include: abstinence; careful choice of sexual partners or monogamous relationships; use of barrier methods of contraception, i.e., diaphragm, condom, cervical cap, etc.; and routine examination.

There is a need for a rapid, inexpensive and widely available test for *Chlamydia trachomatis.*

While oral contraceptives may protect against gonococcal PID, current information does not indicate that oral contraceptives protect against all forms of PID. There are even studies that indicate a two to threefold increase in the prevalence of cervical *Chlamydia trachomatis* infection in oral contraceptive users.

Further Reading

Bump RC. Chlamydia trachomatis as a cause of prepubertal vaginitis. Obstet Gynecol 1985; 65:384–388.

Kane JL, Woodland RM, Forsey T, Darougar S, Elder MG. Evidence of chlamydial infection in infertile women with and without Fallopian tube obstruction. Fertil Steril 1984; 42:843–848.

McCormack WM, Rosner B, McComb DE, Evrard JR, Zinner SH. Infection with Chlamydia trachomatis in female college students. Am J Obstet Gynecol 1985; 121:107–115.

Osborne NG, Pratson L. Sexually transmitted diseases and pregnancy. J Obstet Gynecol Neonat Nurs 1984; 13:9–10.

Osser S, Persson K. Postabortal pelvic infection associated with Chlamydia trachomatis and the influence of humoral immunity. Am J Obstet Gynecol 1984; 150:699–703.

Schaefer C, Harrison HR, Boyce WT, Lewis M. Illnesses in infants born to women with Chlamydia trachomatis infection. Am J Dis Child 1985; 139:127–133.

Shafer MA, Chew KL, Kromhout LK, Beck A, et al. Chlamydial endocervical infections and cytologic findings in sexually active female adolescents. Am J Obstet Gynecol 1985; 151:765–771.

Washington AE, Gove S, Schachter J, Sweet RL. Oral contraceptives, Chlamydia trachomatis infection and pelvic inflammatory disease. J Am Med Assoc 1985; 253:2246–2250.

Uyeda CT, Welborn P, Ellison-Birang N, Shunk K, Tsaouse B. Rapid diagnosis of chlamydial infections with the Microtrak direct test. J Clin Microbiol 1984; 20:948–950.

CONDYLOMATA
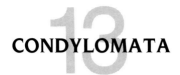

What Are Condylomata?

Condylomata, or venereal warts, are most often sexually transmitted. Hand to genital transmission is rare. These warts are caused by a small DNA virus, a papillomavirus that one cannot start a lab culture from. They are, however, classified according to their types, i.e., human papillovirus DNA Types 6, 11, 16 or 18. These genital warts differ from skin warts. Sexually acquired warts are infectious in about 60 percent of cases; the incubation period is long, from two weeks to eight months, the average being three months.

What Are the Symptoms of Venereal Warts?

Venereal warts usually appear as flat growths in moist areas, usually on the penis, on the vulva or in the vagina or rectum (Figs. 13-1 to 13-5). Cervical, vaginal or anal-rectal warts may go undetected until examined by a physician. It appears that carriers, who do not show outward signs of the infection, may transmit venereal warts.

In fact, the infection may be difficult to detect even in those afflicted. Some physicians believe that most human papillomavirus (HPV) lesions are flat, subclinical proliferations when in the vagina or on the cervix. These can only be seen with colposcopy, a magnification technique that allows the colposcopist to isolate areas of concern for treatment or biopsy.

Even visible lesions are often asymptomatic and painless. They flourish in warm, moist areas and can often be found in association with a discharge or other infections.

In men, they may appear on the glans and shaft of the penis, in the foreskin and its frenulum, in the coronal sulcus or urethral opening, in the anus and rectum, or on the scrotum.

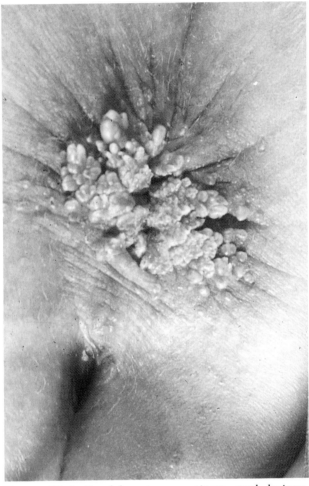

Figure 13–1 Condylomata accuminata—anal lesions. (Reproduced with the permission of The American Academy of Dermatology.)

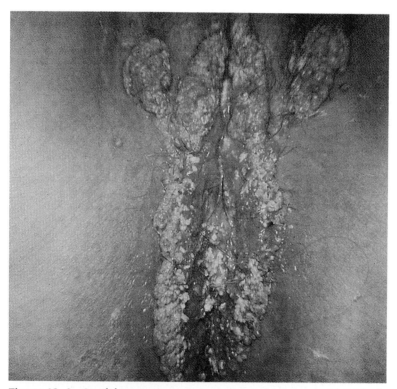

Figure 13-2   Condylomata accuminata—advanced vulvar warts. (With the permission of Schering Corporation, U.S.A.)

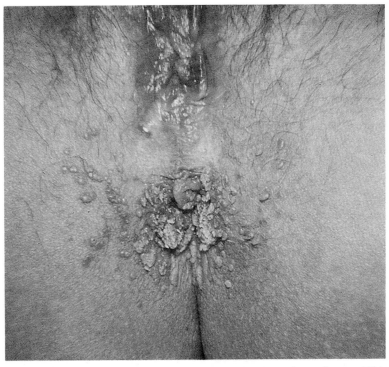

Figure 13–3 Condylomata acccuminata lesions of the vulva and anus. (With the permission of Schering Corporation, U.S.A.)

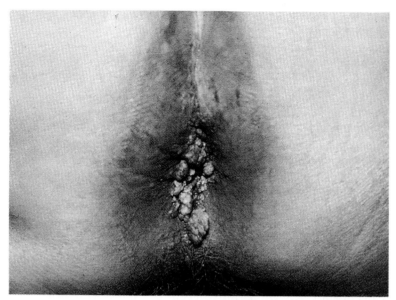

Figure 13-4 Condylomata accuminata—anal-rectal lesions. (With the permission of Schering Corporation, U.S.A.)

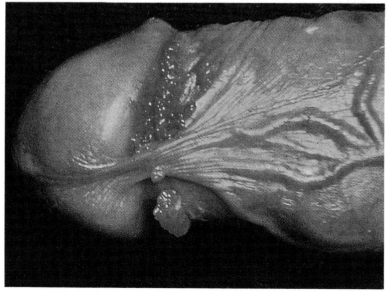

Figure 13-5 Condylomata accuminata—penis. (With the permission of Schering Corporation, U.S.A.)

Anal warts usually occur after anal intercourse but may occur regardless.

In women, the most common sites of infection are the introitus, the opening into the vagina, and the vulva, the labia, but lesions may also be found on the vaginal walls and on the cervix.

How Are HPV Diagnosed?

When lesions are visible, diagnosis by a trained physician is usually quite straightforward. As stated earlier, colposcopy may be necessary to isolate questionable areas of the vagina or cervix that are often reported on PAP smears as cellular atypia.

These lesions must be differentiated from similar-appearing lesions, such as condylomata lata of secondary syphilis, molloscum contagiosum and some benign and malignant tumors.

All patients with condylomata should be checked for concurrent diseases. Up to one-third of women who were initially examined for condylomata have also had one or more additional diseases. Therefore, tests should be done to rule out *Candida albicans*, *Gardnerella vaginalis* and *Chlamydia trachomatis*.

Men should be checked for urethral gonorrhea and nongonococcal urethritis (NGU).

Homosexuals with anal warts are checked via proctoscopy, direct visual examination of the rectal area, for the presence of additional warts and the possibility of rectal gonorrhea.

How Can Condylomata Be Treated?

There are different treatment modalities, including:

1. Podophyllin
2. Cryotherapy with liquid nitrogen
3. Electrical fulguration, i.e., electrocautery
4. CO_2 laser, i.e., carbon dioxide laser
5. Idoxuridine
6. 5-Fluorouracil
7. Trichloroacetic acid

Failure rates are still high with all modalities, so that repeated therapy may be necessary.

Podophyllin

Podophyllin is probably the easiest and most commonly used agent in the treatment of condylomata. It is cytotoxic and can be used between 1 and 3 times per week. It must be washed off within 4 to 5 hours after application; otherwise it can cause serious burns to the area.

The physician applies podophyllin, only because overzealous patients usually apply it too often or leave it on too long. Application of large quantities can cause peripheral neuropathy, damage to the peripheral nerves, as well as coma and hypokalemia, all as a result of lowered potassium levels.

A pregnant woman should not use podophyllin since it may be toxic and so may cause fetal mutations.

Cryotherapy

Cryotherapy using liquid nitrogen has been successful in the treatment of genital warts. For the pregnant woman, it is an acceptable alternative to podophyllin, thus allowing her to avoid a cesarean section or complicated vaginal delivery. Its timely use reduces the risk of transmitting venereal warts to the newborn.

Electrocautery

Electrocautery remains one of the most widely used modalities for the treatment of genital warts. It most often requires general anaesthesia and is primarily used for lesions not treatable by podophyllin, especially those in the vagina and rectum.

CO_2 Laser

Genital warts can be effectively treated with the CO_2 laser. Unfortunately, this modality is not available in all centers as it requires special training and is quite costly to operate. However, this method shows great promise; its use will certainly expand.

Flat condylomata are best treated with the laser. After treatment, 92 percent of patients experience no recurring infection. The laser has also been used in other areas, such as the vagina, urethra, and rectum, with equal success. The advantages of CO_2 laser treatment include: increased precision versus other more traditional modes, minimal damage to surrounding tissue, a controlled depth of penetration, less scarring, reduced pain.

Idoxuridine

Studies seem to indicate that Idoxuridine (IDU) is an effective, nontoxic and inexpensive treatment for genital warts. However, it should probably not be used in pregnancy; when tested, it has induced congenital anomalies in animals.

5-Fluorouracil

Intravaginal therapy with 5-Fluorouracil (5-FU) treatment of Condyloma accuminata, has been as effective as CO_2 treatment. Therefore, 5-FU is more cost effective and does not require a general anesthetic, as does the CO_2 laser. It should not be used on pregnant women.

What Are the Possible Consequences of Genital Warts?

Women suffer the most seriously. There appears to be a link between cervical condylomata and cervical cancer. Condylomata may be involved in the developmental stages of cervical neoplasia, i.e., cancer.

Two distinct types of cervical condylomatous lesions exist:

Human papillomavirus DNA Types 6 and/or 11. These tend to regress spontaneously, or do not recur after treatment, and have virtually no known malignant potential.

Human papillomavirus DNA Types 16 and/or 18. These have a high malignant potential. The association holds true for both cervical and vulvar cancer.

Up to 40 percent of biopsy specimens from 1972 were wrongly diagnosed at that time as early cervical neoplasia, or cancer. When these same specimens were reexamined in 1982, the true diagnosis was found to be cervical condyloma. Since then, diagnostic acumen has greatly improved, and now diagnosis of cervical condyloma or its associated malignancy is more precise.

For years it has been suspected that an infectious agent was involved in the development of human cervical cancer. Investigators have based this conclusion on epidemiological studies. These studies show that the time of first sexual intercourse and the number of sexual partners are the most important factors associated with cervical cancer, and that women whose husbands have had multiple sexual partners are at higher risk of developing cervical cancer.

It is quite clear that a woman's male sexual partners play an important role in the transmission of cervical cancer. As stated earlier, the second wife of a man whose previous wife died of cervical carcinoma runs a greater risk of developing cervical cancer herself.

Other consequences? Infants and young children may develop laryngeal papillomas as a result of being infected by maternal genital warts at delivery. The anal warts of homosexual men have revealed signs of cancer.

Prevention

Condoms.   As is the case with many STDs, using barrier methods of contraception, such as the condom or the diaphragm, will help prevent both the acquisition and spread of venereal warts.

Treatment of Lesions.   Prompt recognition and adequate treatment are necessary to prevent the further spread of disease and the development of precursors to cancer.

Careful Choice of Sexual Partners.   The association of genital warts with cancer seems quite evident. The present lack of proof means that a pragmatic approach to genital warts should be taken nevertheless. Women should have cytology every year, i.e., PAP tests.

Further Reading

Adler MW. Genital warts and molluscum contagiosum. Br Med J 1984; 288:213–215.

Bernstein SG, Voet RL, Guzick DS, et al. Prevalence of papillomavirus infection in colposcopically directed cervical biopsy specimens in 1972 and

1982. Am J Obstet Gynecol 1985; 151:557–581.

Binder MA, Cates GW, Emson HE, et al. The changing concepts of condyloma. Am J Obstet Gynecol 1985; 151:213–219.

Croxson T, Chabon AB, Rorat E, Barash IM. Intraepithelial carcinoma of the anus in homosexual men. Dis Colon Rectum 1984; 27:325–330.

Daling JR, Chu J, Weiss NS, Emel L, Tamini HK. The association of condylomata acuminata and squamous carcinoma of the vulva. Br J Cancer 1984; 50:533–535.

Ferenczy A. Comparison of 5-fluorouracil and CO_2 laser for treatment of vaginal condylomata. Obstet Gynecol 1984; 64:773–778.

SCABIES AND PEDICULOSIS PUBIS

What Are They?

These two ectoparasite infestations are dependent upon the host animal for support, but unlike endoparasites, which live inside the host's body, they infest the outside of the animal. They may be acquired sexually; however, they are by no means always acquired this way. They are usually transmitted person to person but may be transmitted via infected clothing, bedding and, infrequently, in public washrooms.

Scabies

"The itch" is an infestation of the skin by *Sarcoptes scabiei*. This parasite's burrowing habits typically result in an itchy rash with a characteristic distribution or pattern. Scabies were first seen in 1834; the discovery was a real dermatological breakthrough, since at that time it accounted for up to 60 percent of all skin diseases.

The female's burrowing habits prevent it from being seen. As it delves beneath the skin, it deposits eggs, extending its tunnel by 2 mm each day. The larvae hatch and, in order to copulate and continue the cycle, leave the burrow for the surface. Reasons given for the resurgence of scabies in the 1960s and 1980s include: increased sexual promiscuity, increased travel, deteriorating standards of personal hygiene and poor recognition of scabies by medical personnel.

Pediculosis Pubis

There are three types of lice, also commonly known as crabs: head, body and pubic lice. In North America and Western Europe, the incidence of lice has been increasing since the 1960s, and it is now approaching epidemic levels.

The cause of pediculosis pubis is *Phthirus pubis* (Fig. 14-1). The parasite has six legs, four of which terminate in crablike claws that are used to grasp and hold on to body hairs. The parasite's eggs can be seen at the base of the human hair, where they incubate from six to eight days before hatching.

What Are the Symptoms?

Scabies

The most outstanding symptom of scabies is itching—frequently severe and occurring most often at night. At this time, the burrow is quite striking—a thin, greyish line either straight or zigzag, about 2 to 15 mm long. Many other dermatological lesions are associated with scabies. A distinctive feature of this eruption is its distribution: it involves the sides and webs of the fingers; the inner, flexor, aspects of the wrists; the extensor surface of the elbows; the anterior and posterior axillary folds, i.e., the armpits; the skin adjacent to the nipples; the area around

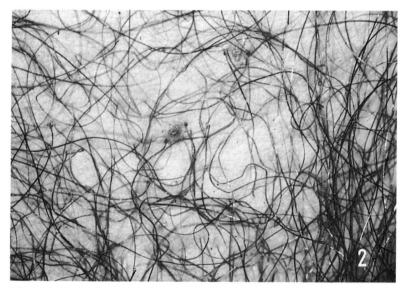

Figure 14–1 Pediculosis pubis–crab-like parasites located in pubic hair. (With the permission of The American Academy of Dermatology.)

the navel; the waist; the penis; the front of the knees, i.e., the extensor surface; and the lower aspects of the feet.

Pediculosis Pubis

Often no symptoms are noticed; however, the pubic area is usually itchy. Occasionally, small, silver flecks can be seen, marking the presence of the parasite or crab. Most often the oval-shaped nits, which are the eggs of the parasite, are cemented to the hair shafts.

How Are Scabies and Lice Diagnosed?

A clinical assessment and direct inspection, with or without a microscope, are all that are required. This is known as diagnosis by recognition.

How Are They Treated?

Both scabies and pubic lice can be treated by topical application, in the form of shampoo, lotion, or cream medication, to kill the mites.

Adults and older children are usually treated with lindane, also known as gamma benzene, commonly seen as hexachloride, Kwell, Kwellada and Scabene. If properly applied, the medication is virtually 100 percent effective. This product may be toxic to the central nervous system if ingested or misused, i.e., too frequently applied. Lindane is still available in Canada without prescription but should be used with caution and probably avoided for infants and very young children. Good alternatives would be crotamiton cream or lotion (Eurax) or 5 percent sulfur precipitate in petroleum.

In order to avoid cross-contamination and reinfection, all members of the family and all sexual contacts should be treated at the same time.

Bedding and clothing should be washed in hot water or dry cleaned immediately after treatment. However, storing outer garments and blankets for two weeks is adequate to get rid of any stray mites; these parasites cannot survive more than a few days away from the skin.

In the case of pediculosis pubis, similar treatment should be repeated in 7 to 10 days to kill lice newly hatched from the surviving eggs. In follow-up treatment, remember to use a fine-toothed comb to pull these away from hair shafts. For nits and parasites in the eyelashes, fine tweezers can be used. Afterwards, apply petroleum jelly to the area.

Following effective treatment, itching may persist for days. Your family physician can prescribe accordingly.

Are There Any Complications Due to Ectoparasites?

Apart from persistent itching after treatment and raised, nodular lesions—symptoms that disappear with time—infestations may also be complicated by scratching. This action may cause secondary bacterial infections that will require prompt medical attention.

How Can Scabies and Pubic Lice Be Prevented?

Proper hygiene, careful choice of sexual partners, as well as awareness and understanding, will lead to early recognition and treatment.

Further Reading

Crissey JT. Scabies and pediculosis pubis. Urol Clin North Am 1984; 11:171–176.
Holmes KK, et al. Sexually transmitted diseases. New York: McGraw-Hill, 1984: 513–517, 517–524.

GONORRHEA

Gonorrhea is a true venereal disease, meaning that it is transmitted from an infected to a noninfected individual by direct personal, usually sexual, contact. The incidence of gonorrhea has increased dramatically since the mid-50s. This can be traced to the introduction of the birth control pill and the IUD, hence the decreased use of more protected forms of contraception—the condom, the diaphragm, and spermicidal preparations. Increased sexual activity has exacerbated the problem. The prevalence of gonorrhea in North America doubled between 1955 and 1981; those in the 15 to 29 age range are at greatest risk of contracting the infection. Up to 60 percent of women who have the infection have no symptoms, compared to 20 percent of men.

The disease has been documented in ancient literature—Chinese, Egyptian, Roman and Greek. Gonorrhea, from the Greek, means "flow of seed." The term was once used to describe the urethral discharge of semen rather than the infectious discharge we now recognize it to be.

Many countries have developed a system of diagnosing and reporting gonorrhea; unfortunately, statistics reflect only reported cases. Many instances are never brought to the attention of health authorities. In the United States, one million cases were reported in 1981. It is estimated that another 1 to 1.5 million were never reported that year.

Gonorrhea is caused by the bacteria *Neisseria gonorrhoeae*, named after the man who first isolated the organism. The organism is easily killed by heat, drying or mild antiseptics. It is not caught from toilet seats or urinals but transmitted from one sexual partner to another through direct contact of one infected mucous membrane with another—via oral, vaginal, urethral, rectal or cervical means.

Although rarely, pussy secretions may be transmitted to other locations, such as the eyes. The bacteria may also spread from the primary sites, causing infection of the uterus, endometritis; the fallopian tubes, salpingitis; the abdominal cavity, peritonitis; the glands of the vulvar area in women, bartholinitis; and the testicles in men, epididymitis.

What Are the Symptoms of Gonorrhea?

In Men.   The incubation period usually extends from three to five days, occasionally longer. There is discomfort, often a burning sensation in the urethra on urination. This may be followed by a urethral discharge that becomes thick, creamy and green yellow in color (Fig. 15-1).

In Women.   There may or may not be abnormal vaginal discharge. There may or may not be a burning sensation on urination. Women who consult their physicians often have symptoms or complaints that relate to a gonococcal infection that has spread upward. Infection of the uterus or fallopian tubes causes abnormal menstrual bleeding and midline lower abdominal pain often, but not always, accompanied by fever and chills.

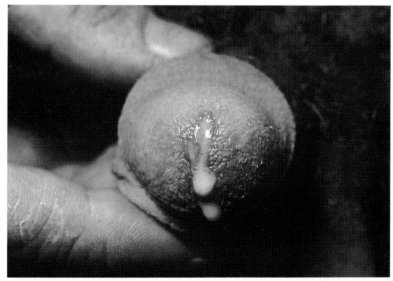

Figure 15–1 Gonorrhea of the urethra with its typically thick, creamy discharge. (With the permission of The American Academy of Dermatology.)

Remember

1.   At least half of infected women have no symptoms.
2.   As compared to noninfected women, women with gonorrhea who use the IUD run a four to eight times greater risk of infection of the fallopian tubes.

In both men and women, if anal intercourse is practiced, possible symptoms of rectal gonorrhea include: increased flatulence, pain on defecation, blood in rectum, mucous-like discharge, warts around the anus, gonorrhea of the pharynx or throat if oral sex is practiced.

Associated Health Risks

Gonorrhea may spread via the bloodstream to other areas of the body. It may lead to problems involving joints, i.e., arthritis, or to skin conditions or inflammation of the heart muscle or lining. The brain tissue may be affected, leading to meningitis, or the liver, resulting in hepatitis. An estimated one percent of cases of mucosal infection will develop into disseminated gonococcal infection (DGI). This is more common in women—80 percent of women with DGI often remain asymptomatic until such complications occur. DGI usually occurs within 7 to 30 days after mucosal involvement, but it has been reported at up to one year after infection. DGI is usually associated with fever in many cases, but not all. Other associated symptoms may include chills, decreased appetite and malaise.

Diagnosis

If any of the symptoms mentioned occur, you should see a physician as soon as possible. Sexual partners should be informed and all further sexual contacts avoided until your doctor declares it safe to resume.

Normally, swabs for culture on special medium are taken from the cervix, the urethra in males, the anal canal and the pharynx. Occasionally, blood tests are taken if DGI is suspected, but there is no specific blood test for Neisseria gonorrhoeae.

Treatment

Gonorrhea is treated effectively by antibiotics administered orally or intramuscularly and, at times, intravenously. In the past, penicillin was always the drug of choice, but in the past decade gonorrhea strains resistant to penicillin have been emerging. Treatment regimes have changed accordingly.

Partners of gonorrhea-positive individuals should be treated whether or not their cultures are positive.

Complications of Gonorrhea

DGI. See page 161.

Pelvic Inflammatory Disease. As a complication of gonorrhea, this is common in women. The organism spreads to the uterus and through the fallopian tubes into the pelvic area. This condition may require hospitalization and is known to result in blockage of fallopian tubes and subsequent sterility.

Ectopic Pregnancy. An ectopic pregnancy is one situated outside the uterus. A sperm fertilizes an egg, and because of damage to the fallopian tubes, the fertilized egg cannot find its way to the uterus. It starts to divide, and the fetus develops. A fetus cannot survive outside the uterus, and the developing placenta may damage surrounding tissue, causing internal hemorrhage. Therefore, an ectopic pregnancy must be terminated by surgical removal. It is not a viable pregnancy and it may endanger the mother.

From 1971 to 1978, ectopic pregnancies increased by 53 percent, reflecting an increasing incidence of PIDs.

Conditions in Newborns. Ophthalmia neonatorium, an eye infection in newborns, continues to cause concern. Silver nitrate is used at birth to prevent such a condition, yet still 1.9 percent of infants born to mothers who have gonorrhea will develop ophthalmia neonatorium.

The pregnancies of women with gonorrhea also show an increased incidence of prematurity: premature rupture of fetal membranes and intrauterine growth retardation of the fetus.

Prevention

This is achieved through:

1. Careful selection of sexual partners

2. Avoidance of unprotected sex with new partners—i.e., use of a condom, diaphragm and spermicidal preparations
3. Restricting the number of sexual partners
4. Regular cultures of those at risk of infection, i.e., prostitutes and other sexually active individuals, thus decreasing the number of infections transmitted
5. Prophylactic treatment with antibiotics, without benefit of culture-positive results, in the event of possible contact with an infected person; hence, avoiding complications in asymptomatic individuals and also controlling the spread of infection

Further Reading

Al-Suleiman SA, Grimes EM, Jonas HS. Disseminated gonococcal infections. Obstet Gynecol 1983; 61:48–51.

Fraser JJ, Rettig PJ, Kaplan DW. Prevalence of cervical Chlamydia trachomatis and Neisseria gonorrhoeae in female adolescents. Pediatrics 1983; 71:333–336.

Handsfield HH. Gonorrhea and uncomplicated gonococcal infection. In: Holmes KK, et al, eds. Sexually transmitted diseases. New York: McGraw-Hill, 1984; 205–220.

Lutz B, Mogabgab WJ, Parks D, et al. Comparison of ceftizoxime and penicillin for the treatment of uncomplicated gonorrhea. J Antimicrob Chemother 1982; 10, Suppl. C:229–235.

SYPHILIS

The Italians called it "the French disease" or "the Spanish disease"; the French called it "the Neopolitan sickness"; the English called it "the French disease", and the Scots called it "grandgor," or the "Neopolitan sickness". As with many sexually transmitted diseases, every group wants to blame some other source for this unwelcome introduction into the community.

Syphilis was epidemic in the late fifteenth century. The disease got its name from a poem by Fracastorius, written in 1530, about an afflicted shepherd named Syphilus. Since the disease appeared in Europe at the time when Columbus was returning from the West Indies, Europeans felt it had been imported from America.

To complicate matters, wars have always fueled the spread of this disease, given the movement of troops and increased sexual encounters in times of conflict. Biblical and early Chinese writings described the cutaneous manifestations of syphilis long before any record of the disease in the Americas appeared.

Most cases of syphilis occur in the most sexually active age group, those who are 20 to 39 years of age. Fifty-four percent of primary and secondary syphilis cases in 1980 in the United Kingdom were contracted by homosexuals.

A patient who has been infected with syphilis endangers, on average, three sexual partners. Aggressive contact tracing and epidemiological treatment of all recently exposed persons are the most important steps in controlling syphilis, or any other STD.

What Is Syphilis?

The microorganism responsible for syphilis is bacterial in nature and is known as *Treponema pallidum*, of the order *Spirochaeta*. Since 1965, as a result of the widespread use of antibiotics, there has been a decline in the incidence of the disease among heterosexuals. But syphilis was not as manageable among homosexuals, not until AIDS forced many to change their sexual habits and thus reduce the incidence of many STDs in their community.

How Does One Get Syphilis?

Syphilis is passed from an infectious person to a new host when, during sexual intercourse, the mucosal lesions contact the moist, mucosal surfaces of the sexual partner. The peak incidence of syphilis occurs between the ages of 20 and 24. The obvious exception to contracting the disease through intercourse is congenital syphilis, whereby the newborn innocently acquires the infection via the placenta.

What Are the Symptoms?

Syphilis is divided into four phases:

Primary. The incubation period is about 21 days. Chancres (Figs. 16-1, 16-2), usually painless, appear on affected areas; if left untreated, the chancres will heal spontaneously in 10 to 90 days, the average time span being 3 weeks. Lymph-node swelling in the affected region usually accompanies this lesion. Lesions that appear in areas other than the genitalia may have an atypical appearance. The affected areas usually include the penis and the vulva.

Secondary. This period is characterized by a rash and generalized enlargement of the lymph nodes. In most cases, the secondary phase starts within a few weeks or months after primary lesions have disappeared. Other symptoms may include general malaise, fever, sore throat, headache, skin or mucosal manifestations, patchy hair loss and, in some, liver involvement, i.e., hepatitis.

Latent. The latent period is symptom-free and may last for several years. Serology, blood tests, will be positive, however.

Late Syphilis and Neurosyphilis. Tertiary syphilis may occur as early as five years after the onset of an untreated infection. The principle morbidity and mortality of syphilis result largely from manifestations of illness in the skin, bones, central

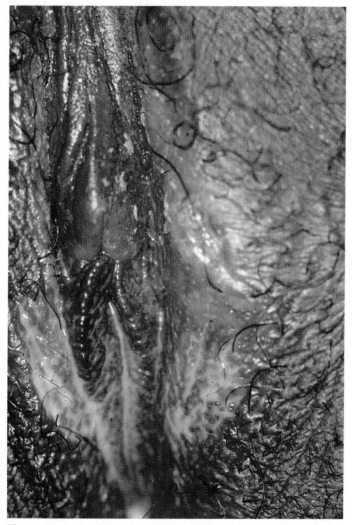

Figure 16–1 Syphilis-primary lesion of the vulva. (With permission of The American Academy of Dermatology.)

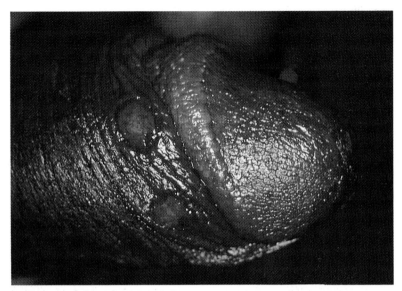

Figure 16–2 Syphilis–primary lesion of the penis. (With permission of The American Academy of Dermatology.)

nervous system and viscera, particularly in the heart and great vessels.

Neurosyphilis may manifest itself in personality changes, eye changes, delusions and hallucinations, intellectual deterioration and abnormal speech, seizures, headaches, insomnia, confusion and disorientation.

What Are the Associated Health Risks?

As previously mentioned, syphilis in its later stages may involve most any organ system, causing devastation if left untreated.

Neurosyphilis will leave its victims permanently incapacitated. Antibiotic therapy may clear the body of the infective organisms, but structural damage to the nervous system, in the late stages of the disease, are irreversible. In the case of paresis, partial paralysis, treatment may not stop the condition from progressing.

Today, cardiovascular syphilis is no longer common. However, it may appear in late syphilis as an aortic aneurysm, the dilatation of the aorta. The aneurysm may rupture and cause death, coronary artery disease or aortic valve disease.

Infants who have contracted congenital syphilis are usually born without signs of the disease; routine screening of blood is carried out to isolate these cases.

Since syphilis is no longer commonly seen in most countries, and since routine serology is performed on all pregnant mothers and their newborns, the serious complications associated with the disease are usually avoided.

How Is Syphilis Diagnosed?

The well-known blood test for VD, called VDRL, is widely used to screen segments of the population. It detects syphilis only; no other STD can be diagnosed with this test.

Typically, when a VDRL is requested, blood is tested in many different ways before an accurate diagnosis is reached, i.e., the VDRL slide test, the FTA-ABS test and the MHA-TP test. These blood tests should be carried out on people who are likely to have had multiple sex partners within short periods of time, such as male and female prostitutes, homosexuals attending bath houses and patients seen for STDs other than syphilis. Since a fetus can be infected, all pregnant women should be routinely screened to prevent congenital syphilis. Women at risk should be rescreened later in pregnancy.

If patients are suspected of having neurosyphilis, then lumbar puncture and examination of cerebrospinal fluids (CSF) are necessary.

How Is Syphilis Treated?

Treatment varies according to the stage of the disease. Penicillin remains the drug of choice, but equally effective medication is available for patients with penicillin allergies. Early treatment of syphilis in pregnancy can prevent neurosyphilis in the newborn.

Prevention

This is achieved through:

1. Regular screening of individuals at risk, i.e., those with multiple partners
2. Avoiding unprotected sex
3. Carefully selecting partners - the fewer, the better
4. Avoiding sexual contact if being treated for syphilis, until your physician advises that intercourse is safe

Further Reading

Holmes KK, Mardh PA, Sparling PF, Wiesner PJ. Sexually transmitted diseases. New York: McGraw-HIll, 1984: 298–305, 305–313, 313–318, 318–334, 352–374, 374–385.

Sacks SL. Genital ulcers—syphilis, herpes, and chancroid. Med N Am, Infect 2, 1983. 526–527.

VIRAL HEPATITIS

What Is Viral Hepatitis?

This is a common, infectious disease caused by one of several viruses that attack the liver. It often results in a clinical syndrome known as jaundice.

Three types of viral hepatitis have been observed: hepatitis A, hepatitis B and non-A, non-B hepatitis.

Traditionally, hepatitis infections have not been regarded as sexually transmitted diseases, and indeed very often they are not. However, as we come to understand changing sexual practices, it becomes apparent that sexual transmission of these viral agents has become more and more common.

Each year in the United States approximately 200,000 hepatitis B infections occur. Chronic carriers may make up as many as 10 percent of adult cases. In Canada, 20,000 cases of hepatitis B occurred in 1985.

How Does One Get Hepatitis?

Hepatitis A

Hepatitis A is generally known as infectious hepatitis. It is caused by a virus usually excreted in the feces. A person has either had direct contact with recently infected stool, i.e., through oral-genital or oral-anal contact, or indirect fecal contact has contaminated hands, eating utensils, dishes or water supplies. Drinking water and food contamination by hepatitis A virus may cause an epidemic.

No chronic carrier state for hepatitis A virus has ever been demonstrated; that is to say, that after an acute illness, no hepatitis A sufferers become chronic carriers of that antigen.

In Europe and North America, the prevalence of infectious hepatitis has fallen in recent decades because of improved sanitation. Only one-third of the United States population has anti-hepatitis A virus antibodies—which indicates previous exposure to the hepatitis A antigen—in contrast to a prevalence of about 95 percent in underdeveloped countries.

Hepatitis B

Hepatitis B is commonly known as serum hepatitis. It is found in virtually all body fluids and secretions of infected individuals. As well as being transmitted sexually, it may be passed through blood transfusions, through mucous membrane exposure to the virus or through puncturing of the skin by contaminated instruments. Ear piercing, tattooing, and the "dirty needles" used by drug addicts are possible vehicles of transmission.

Blood containing hepatitis B virus is highly infectious; however, blood is not the only body fluid containing hepatitis B. Although other fluids may not be as contagious, they can still transmit the virus.

Sexual transmission will occur through oral ingestion of ejaculate or fecal ingestion in oral-genital or oral-anal sex. Rectal intercourse among homosexuals is also responsible for transmission of the hepatitis B virus. Hepatitis B tends to be a more serious condition than hepatitis A, accounting for 535 deaths in Canada in 1978.

Transmission of hepatitis B occurs not only from ill patients, but from the estimated worldwide 5 to 15 percent of disease carriers. This carrier state of hepatitis B is the major health problem associated with the virus. In North America, northern Europe, western Europe and parts of Australia, less than 0.1 percent of the population carry markers, i.e., antigens or antibodies of the hepatitis B virus (5.5 percent of male homosexuals). In other areas, 1 to 5 percent are carriers; in still other areas, 10 percent; and in tropical Africa, the Pacific Islands and particularly along the coast of China, 10 to 35 percent of the population carry markers of hepatitis B virus in their circulation. Sexual promiscuity is associated with higher carrier rates.

More than 50 percent of hepatitis B cases are transmitted through direct physical, often sexual, contact; 33 percent of those infected are homosexuals. The predominance of the disease among the homosexual population relates to contact with various different sexual partners, as well as personal sexual practices, including anal-genital intercourse and anilingus, anal-oral intercourse.

Feces and anorectal mucosa may often contain infectious hepatitis B virus. Fragile, bleeding rectal mucosa may be particularly susceptible to infection from hepatitis virus contained in saliva or semen.

Because hepatitis B virus has been detected in saliva, tears, nasal washings, menstrual blood, vaginal secretions and semen, many potential routes for infection obviously exist.

Non-A, Non-B Hepatitis

This third type of hepatitis is caused by one or many viruses other than A or B. Blood transfusion is the major known route of infection. Studies of acute cases of viral hepatitis occurring in potentially sexually active 15- to 44-year-olds indicate that almost 50 percent are Type B, 20 to 25 percent are Type A and 20 to 25 percent are non-A, non-B.

What Are the Symptoms of Hepatitis?

Typically, acute viral hepatitis passes through many phases. The first is an asymptomatic incubation period.

Hepatitis A: 2 to 6 weeks
Hepatitis B: 1 to 4 months
Non-A, Non-B: 50 days on average

The second phase lasts one week and is the prodromal or prejaundice phase, with symptoms such as lack of appetite, nausea, occasional vomiting, headache, malaise, fatigue, and a distaste for cigarettes, coffee, and tea.

The third phase is the jaundice phase. By then, the urine has darkened, and the stool has become lighter in color, almost pasty. The liver frequently becomes enlarged.

Viral hepatitis may last a few weeks; full recovery may take a few months. In 10 percent of patients, a relapse occurs. Fulminant hepatitis occurs in less than one percent of those affected and often leads to death. Note that acute viral hepatitis is not always apparent; there may be no symptoms or signs. Yet, these seemingly healthy people remain infectious.

Jaundice may occur in only one of four patients. In most patients, hepatitis is a self-limiting condition; that is, one that resolves itself without further risk of transmission or complication. However, about 6 to 10 percent of patients with hepatitis B fail to clear the infection within six months; these are chronic hepatitis B antigen, HBAg, carriers. They have the most long-term complications of hepatitis B, including cirrhosis and hepatocellular cancer of the liver.

Manifestations of hepatitis B situated or originating outside the liver have been well documented, including arthralgias, or joint pain; skin rash; arthritis; pleurisy; kidney involvement, or glomerulonephritis; and neurological involvement, Guillain-Barré Syndrome.

How Is Hepatitis Diagnosed?

A physician, equipped with a good medical history of the patient, as well as data from a thorough examination, can often make a diagnosis. Typing of hepatitis is done through blood tests that measure specific antigen and antibody.

The course of the disease is carefully monitored through liver function tests, i.e., blood tests. These blood tests usually demonstrate three responses:

1. Transient antigen or self-limiting disease in 70 percent of affected individuals; i.e., Ag positive becomes Ag negative
2. Antibody presence without documented antigen, i.e., evidence of past infection, which occurs in less than 25 percent of cases; patients have usually had hepatitis B but were never ill; i.e., Ab positive without ever having the documented Ag
3. Persistent antigen chronic hepatitis B (only) carrier—5 percent along with antibody; these people recover from initial contact; they may not have been ill but they continue to be contagious; i.e., Ag positive, and Ab positive persists after the disease has passed

What Are the Possible Consequences of Hepatitis?

As already noted, hepatitis is usually a self-limiting disease. The greatest threat in carriers of hepatitis B, is excretion of the virus well after the clinical illness has past. The hepatitis B virus can also still contribute to permanent liver damage in the form of chronic hepatitis or fulminant, life-threatening hepatitis.

Chronic, active hepatitis develops in 5 to 10 percent of those with clinically diagnosed hepatitis B. According to a study done in New York by Drs. Szmuness and Stevens, HBAg carrier ratios were 0.2 percent among white blood donors, 5.5 percent among male homosexuals and about 9 percent among people of Chinese extraction. Higher carrier ratios were found among the institutionalized and the sexually promiscuous.

Carriers of chronic hepatitis B may transmit the disease to the newborn. In the United States, about 5 percent of children born to HBAg positive mothers became positive themselves by the end of their first year of life. Patients with chronic hepatitis may go on to develop cirrhosis and, rarely, hepatocellular cancer of the liver.

How Is Hepatitis Treated?

At this time, there is no specific treatment for hepatitis infections. Rest, adequate diet and avoidance of liver irritants such as alcohol are generally recommended.

How Can Hepatitis Be Avoided?

Infected individuals should avoid intimate contact with others until antigen is no longer being excreted. Likewise, food handlers should not be on the job until they are no longer excreting the virus.

Individuals who become chronic carriers of hepatitis B should be properly instructed as to their status, and should probably advise sexual partners of the possibility of transmission.

Passive Protective Immunization

Hepatitis A

Passive immunity, that which occurs when antibodies from a donor pool are used, can be achieved through the intramuscular injection of immune serum globulin, gammaglobulin. This immunity is short-lived. The serum is usually given to family contacts of patients with hepatitis A or to individuals traveling to developing countries, the goal being to limit epidemics in closed communities.

Hepatitis B

Passive immunization can be achieved by injecting hepatitis B immune globulin, derived from plasma obtained from a donor pool, with a high concentration of hepatitis B antibodies. This serum is recommended for patients at high risk of contracting hepatitis B, namely:

1. Patients who have possibly received contaminated blood transfusions
2. Hospital staff at high risk because of recent exposure to the blood or secretions of patients with proven hepatitis B infection, i.e., via a pin prick or contamination of the mucous membranes of the eyes
3. Those who have recently had sexual contact with proven HBAg carriers

Active Immunization

In the absence of any safe treatment for those in an antigen carrier state, the most promising way to prevent hepatitis B is through long-lasting protective immunization.

A vaccine for hepatitis B now exists. Since the virus cannot be grown independently, it is isolated from the blood of chronically infected but asymptomatic carriers, i.e., antigen carriers. When administered to these same carriers, this vaccine does not eradicate the carrier state. Its potential lies in its ability to immunize individuals who have not yet been exposed to hepatitis B but who are at greatest risk of contracting the infection, whether under sexual or occupational conditions. The vaccine is 95 to 100 percent successful and is free of significant side effects.

Appropriate target groups include male homosexuals with multiple partners, intravenous drug abusers, patients and staff in institutions for the mentally retarded, health care workers who come into contact with blood or other infected material, patients and staff in dialysis units, recipients of certain blood products, household contacts of hepatitis B carriers, and other, special high-risk populations like prostitutes.

Of special interest is the immunization, with this vaccine, of newborns born to hepatitis B antigen carrier mothers.

Procedures for the manufacture of hepatitis B vaccine are effective in deactivating viruses in every known group, including those with the AIDS virus. In other words, the vaccine is safe.

Each year in the United States, there are about 200,000 new cases of hepatitis B. Up to 1,000 die with fulminant hepatitis, and 10,000 to 20,000 experience chronic hepatitis B. An estimated half of these cases of hepatitis B could be prevented by immunizing all persons who are at high risk of contracting the virus.

Further Reading

Beasley RP, Hwang LY, Lin CC, Ko YC, Twu SJ. Incidence of hepatitis among students at a university in Taiwan. Am J Epidemiol 1983; 117:213–222.

Gerety RJ, Tabor E. Newly licensed hepatitis B vaccine. J Am Med Assoc 1983; 249:745–746.

Goldstein J. Concurrent acute infection with hepatitis A and B. J Am Med Assoc 1983; 249:727–728.

Howell DR, Barbara AJ. How many people become carriers after infection with HBV? Vox Sang 1983; 44:121–122.

Lemon SM. Viral hepatitis. In: Holmes KK, et al, eds. Sexually transmitted diseases. New York: McGraw-Hill, 1984.

Macek C. AIDS transmission: what about the hepatitis B vaccine? J Am Med Assoc 1983; 249:685–686.

VAGINITIS

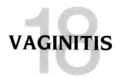

The most common gynecological complaint of young sexually active women is that of abnormal vaginal discharge. Such a discharge may be normal for some, but it is often an important symptom of vaginal infection. It may or may not be sexually acquired but can be sexually transmitted to a partner. Vaginal discharge may accompany not only vaginal infections but also cervical, endometrial infections, as well as infections of the fallopian tubes. When vulvar or cervical tissues are involved, the condition is called vulvitis or cervicitis. A nondiseased but infected carrier may transmit these infections to a susceptible host.

Symptoms vary according to the specific organisms involved. The most common symptoms include:

1. Abnormal vaginal discharge
2. Vaginal or vulvar itching or pain
3. Foul-smelling discharge
4. Reddened and swollen area
5. Pain during intercourse or urination
6. Fever and abdominal pain if associated with infection elsewhere

The vagina is the ideal environment for the growth of certain organisms. It is a warm and moist environment with its own normal flora and conditions that usually discourage the growth of invading organisms. However, the environment may be altered and thus becomes susceptible to infection.

Various general diseases predispose the vagina to infection. For example, pregnancy and diabetes change vaginal secretions, allowing pathogenic, or abnormal, organisms to grow.

Foreign bodies, such as contraceptive devices or tampons left in too long, as well as irritating chemical douches, may cause vaginitis. The birth control pill may effect changes in the vaginal environment, much like pregnancy, that will enable fungal infections to establish themselves more readily.

Other factors thought to contribute to vaginal infections include: tight-fitting clothes, frequent douching, highly perfumed soaps, douches or bubble baths and synthetic undergarments.

Serious, long-term physical consequences of vaginitis are very uncommon, even though discomfort may be intense. The condition is regarded as more of a nuisance than anything else.

Still, vaginitis merits consideration, and it is best to present the most common causative agents of vaginal, vulvar, and cervical infection separately.

Candida Albicans

Candida albicans accounts for the majority of clinical, vaginal yeast infections. It is probably responsible for 60 to 80 percent of vaginitis cases. The incidence of *Candida albicans* increased fourfold from 1944 to 1976.

The infection commonly inhabits the mouth and the bowel, i.e., the large intestine and the vagina in 20 to 50 percent of healthy individuals. For many, it is a normal organism living in harmony with its host; this is called a commensal. However, since *Candida albicans* may later cause disease in this host if certain conditions for growth are met, or if the host's defense is weakened in some way, the infection is also known as an opportunistic pathogen. As previously discussed, pregnancy and diabetes may foster the disease; change in vaginal flora following antibiotic therapy may also make it easy for infection to develop. Similarly, when one's immune system is compromised, as in the case with AIDS victims or patients undergoing cancer therapy, they may be affected by this opportunistic organism.

Clinical Disease

Vulvovaginitis is the most common clinical manifestation of candidial infection. Such infection is usually acute. It may also become chronic and recur frequently. Symptoms and signs of the infection may include:

1. Vulvar itching
2. Vulvar, vaginal and cervical erythema, redness
3. Vaginal discharge ranging from scant to a thick, white, curdlike material

4. Possible external pain on urination as the urine passes over the inflamed, external genitalia
5. Pain on intercourse
6. Infection more severe just prior to menstruation; as menstrual flow becomes established, symptoms subside

Male partners of women suffering from vulvovaginitis may complain of itching or of atypical inflammation of the glans penis. These conditions occur most often in an uncircumcised man. Most men, even if exposed to the organism, show no clinical signs of the infection.

Candida albicans may be transmitted to the newborn. Its most common manifestation is thrush, oral candidiasis.

Diagnosis

A physician can make a clinical diagnosis in an office setting, and treatment can be initiated prior to receiving confirmation from vaginal swabs sent for lab culture. Wet mounts can also be prepared, allowing the examiner to identify the organism under a microscope.

Treatment

Modalities differ from one clinic to another. It is not necessary to treat incidental findings of *Candida* in asymptomatic patients. It may not even be necessary to treat a male partner in the event that the female partner has an acute infection. Some physicians may wait to see if recurrent infection occurs before treating the man, while some would treat both man and woman.

Abstinence is advisable during the treatment period to allow for healing of the damaged lining of the vagina. It is probably safe to have intercourse as soon as pain or discomfort subsides.

Treatment usually involves the vaginal application of cream, ovules, suppositories or medicated tampons for one to ten days, depending on the treatment modality used. There are a large number of preparations available; all are effective in eradicating most vaginal infections produced by *Candida albicans*. Occasionally, oral preparations of mycostatin are needed for subsequent infections.

Trichomonas Vaginalis

Trichomonas vaginalis is a protozoan organism. Of its group, it is the only one to inhabit the human urogenital tract. Unlike *Gardnerella* infections and *Candida*, which may be acquired without sexual contact—though often transmitted sexually—Trichomonal vaginitis is the only vaginitis that can be described as an STD. It is neither a normal commensal nor an opportunistic organism. Its presence means infection has occurred.

As symptoms in men are uncommon, it is easily spread, quite unknowingly, from male sexual partners to other women. Nevertheless, existing data suggest that the prevalence of this disease is decreasing.

Trichomonas vaginalis may survive outside the body, on toilet seats, for example, although its infectiousness outside the body has not been documented. Nonsexual transmission may, therefore, occur, but it is felt to be a rare event.

Clinical Disease

The *Trichomonas vaginalis* organism causes trichomoniasis. When found in the vagina, the infection usually comes complete with symptoms. There may be increased vaginal secretions that are yellow green, frothy and malodorous, but most often the symptoms are not so dramatic. They include vulvar itching and burning on urination over the genital area affected. As with candidal infections, symptoms often diminish with menstruation. In fact, forty percent of these infections have no concomitant symptoms and may be found on routine examination.

Trichomonas vaginalis will cause infections in men—usually they are asymptomatic. Infrequently, it causes urethritis, inflammation of the urethra, along with discharge and/or burning on urination. Most commonly, the possibility of such infection is only conceded after treatment for nonspecific urethritis has failed. In such cases the physician probably attempted to eradicate a nongonococcal infection with broad-spectrum antibiotics. *Trichomonas vaginalis* also causes infection of the prostate, known as prostatis; the penis, balanitis; and the epididymis, epididymitis. Stricture or abnormal narrowing of the urethra, has also been reported.

Diagnosis

Clinical diagnosis may be made and treatment initiated prior to confirmation by culture or wet mount.

Treatment

Metronidazole, brand name Flagyl, is the only effective oral treatment available for *Trichomonas vaginalis*. Different modalities allow for treatments in one dose or in regimens of up to 1 week. Partners are usually treated concurrently. The antibiotic may cause nausea and vomiting, and alcohol consumption may exaggerate this response in many people, causing them to be violently ill.

Unlike the treatment procedure for *Candida*, it is strongly recommended that asymptomatic, infected females be treated in order to prevent further transmission of the disease.

Metronidazole is not recommended for pregnant women, and breast feeding should be interrupted for 24 hours after its ingestion.

Gardnerella Vaginalis

Gardnerella vaginalis, once known as *Hemophilus vaginalis*, is a bacterial organism found to be associated with abnormal vaginal discharge. In asymptomatic females, it is considered either a commensal or an opportunistic organism, much as *Candida* is. It has also been linked with a disease known as nonspecific vaginitis. Our understanding of *Gardnerella* is incomplete; therefore, recognition and treatment are often controversial.

The fishlike odor in patients infected by the *Gardnerella* organism is caused by a group of anaerobic bacteria that operate in conjunction with *Gardnerella*.

On routine screening, 68 percent of women show evidence of *Gardnerella vaginalis*, without evidence of vaginal disease per se.

Clinical Manifestations

Women with *Gardnerella*-associated vaginitis may complain of a mild to moderate discharge that is gray, homogenous and odiferous. Vulvar symptoms are usually milder than those related to *Trichomonas* or *Candida*. The secretions tend to have a "fishy" odor, derived from the amines liberated by the anaerobic organisms described earlier. The odor may be particularly offensive during menstruation and after intercourse.

Infection outside the vagina may occur, as the organism may travel to the bloodstream after abortions or delivery. *Gardnerella vaginalis* may also infect the newborn.

Diagnosis

Clinical diagnosis as well as cultures and wet mounts are used.

Treatment

Metronidazole is the drug of choice, yet it is probably best not to treat the organisms if they are found in healthy, asymptomatic individuals. To date, there does not seem to be any reason to treat sexual partners.

Recurrence of vaginal infections are common. As a rule, they have no significant, long-term physical consequences.

Cervicitis

Occasionally, discharge may result from an infection of the cervix, cervicitis, by *Chlamydia trachomatis*, gonorrhea or herpes simplex virus, *Trichomonas*, *Gardnerella* or condylomata, the genital warts described earlier. These cervical infections often have no significant symptoms and are only found during routine annual exams. Often cervicitis will be recognized only after the infection has spread, causing deep pain on intercourse, lower abdominal pain, bleeding after intercourse, midcycle bleeding—not to be confused with the breakthrough bleeding associated with the pill—and unusually heavy periods.

Appropriate cultures will help to pinpoint a causative agent; treatment can then be initiated.

Prevention

All vaginal infections can be prevented through reducing the risk of exposure by reducing the number of sexual partners—preferably to one. New sexual partners should use condoms as well as spermicidal gels before genital contact.

Once a stable relationship becomes established, other forms of contraception may be used with less risk of vaginal infection developing.

NONGONOCOCCAL URETHRITIS (NONSPECIFIC URETHRITIS)

Nongonococcal urethritis (NGU) or nonspecific urethritis (NSU) are names given to infections of the urethra, usually in men, that are not caused by gonorrhea. These infections are usually sexually transmitted, although similar symptoms may result from using certain irritants, such as highly perfumed soaps. Urethritis is four times as common as gonorrhea. Among the organisms considered responsible for the condition are *Chlamydia*, responsible for 40 to 50 percent of cases, and *Trichomonas*, 3 to 5 percent of cases. Women may have urethral symptoms similar to men's, but this is not common.

NGU is epidemic in North America and Europe. Since this condition is not reportable by physicians to public health agencies in Canada and the United States, it is difficult to accurately assess. NGU usually appears in men within 7 to 21 days after sexual contact with an infected partner. The possibility of unknowingly transmitting the organisms to other partners in the interim is a real problem; *Chlamydia*, for example, is more often than not asymptomatic in men and women.

What Are the Symptoms of NGU?

Typically, a man arrives at a clinic complaining of urethral discharge and a burning sensation on urination. The discharge is often pronounced in the morning and is usually scanty and clear, except in some cases of *Trichomonas*, whereby it will be greenish in color. Often symptoms are so mild as to be ignored. Yet such untreated cases remain an important health problem; they increase the risk of further spread.

The most common symptoms reported are:

1. Painful urination

2. Urethral discharge
3. Itchy feeling in the urethra
4. Urgent need to urinate
5. Heaviness in the genitalia
6. Persistent discomfort in the urethra between urinations

What Organisms Can Cause NGU?

1. *Chlamydia*, in up to 60 percent of cases
2. *Trichomonas*, 5 percent incidence
3. *Gardnerella*, less than 1 percent incidence
4. *Candida*
5. Herpes

Diagnosis

Culture mediums are used to identify most organisms; however, no mediums are commercially available for *Chlamydia*. Common diagnostic tools include:

1. For *Chlamydia*: immunofluorescence technique (Microtrak)
2. For *Trichomonas*: culture and wet mount
3. For *Candida*: culture wet mount
4. For herpes: viral cultures

Treatment

This varies according to the organism suspected. It has become more and more common, when gonorrhea or *Chlamydia* are suspected as possible pathogens in urethritis, to treat patients with a regime that may eradicate both organisms. Tetracycline and its derivatives are the drugs of choice. If cultures indicate gonorrhea, the disease may be resistant to conventional drug therapy. Alternative therapy may be necessary. It should be reiterated that urethritis may be caused by gonorrhea, i.e., gonococcal urethritis and non gonorrhea organisms, i.e., nongonococcal urethritis (NGU) or nonspecific urethritis (NSU).

Complications in Men

Conditions related to urethritis, whereby organisms ascend

into the lower urinary tract, may include infections of the epididymis or prostate.

Epididymitis is a painful condition in the scrotal sac. There is usually some swelling and occasionally some redness. Most commonly, epididymitis is caused by gonorrhea or a nongonococcal organism such as *Chlamydia.*

Prostatitis is a painful condition of the prostate, causing swelling and occasional discharge and low back pain. A rectal exam usually confirms the diagnosis; treatment for gonorrhea or *Chlamydia* is then initiated. Occasionally, chronic prostatitis occurs.

Too frequently the significance of NGU or NSU is not stressed to male patients. NGU, or NSU, is an STD just as gonorrhea is. If it is not promptly treated, the condition will spread, and because it does not produce symptoms in many men and often causes symptom-free conditions in most women, serious complications such as sterility or pelvic inflammatory disease may ensue.

Men being treated should avoid all sexual contact from the first sign of symptoms until they are cleared by their physicians. While they are taking antibiotics, they should remember that they may still be infectious. They should advise sexual contacts of their condition so that their partners may also see their physicians for evaluation and treatment.

All prescribed medication should be taken in order to eradicate the organism. Too often medication is discontinued as soon as symptoms subside, in which case the infection will recur. Eventually, strains of organisms resistant to the prescribed medication could develop.

Further Reading

Bowie WR, et al. Bacteriology of the urethra in normal men and men with nongonococcal urethritis. J Clin Microbiol 1977; 6:482.

Bowmer MI. Urethritis and epididymitis. Med N Am, Infect 2, 1983; 499–505.

Dunlop EMC, et al. Chlamydial infection. Incidence of "nonspecific" urethritis. Br J Vener Dis 1972; 48:425.

Kuberski T. Trichomonas vaginalis associated with nongonococcal urethritis and prostatitis. Sex Transm Dis 1980; 7:135.

McChesney JA, et al. Acute urethritis in male college students. J Am Med Assoc 1973; 226:37.

Wong JL, et al. The etiology of nongonococcal urethritis in men attending a venereal disease clinic. Sex Transm Dis 1977; 4:4.

PELVIC INFLAMMATORY DISEASE

Bacterial organisms known to infect the cervix may migrate upward into the uterus and through the fallopian tubes, causing a condition known as pelvic inflammatory disease. In women, this is the most serious common manifestation of sexually transmitted disease. The organisms usually implicated are gonorrhea, and *Chlamydia*. *Chlamydia* is the most frequent causative agent of STDs in the developed world. It has been isolated in up to 35 percent of cases of confirmed salpingitis or pelvic inflammatory disease (PID).

PID may sometimes result from a complication of abortion.

The highest rate of PIDs occurs in females between the ages of 15 and 20, reflecting the fact that women are experiencing initial sexual encounters at an increasingly younger age. A woman with two or more sexual partners has a 4.5 times greater chance of developing PID than a woman with one partner. Twenty percent of women with PID have subsequent attacks.

An estimated 10 to 17 percent of women with untreated gonorrhea will develop PID. The span of time between acquiring the gonococcal bacterium and developing PID is short.

PID is three to four times more common in women with IUDs. In addition, a woman who has never borne a child and who has an IUD, has a seven to nine times greater risk of PID than a woman who has had a child and is using an IUD. Twenty percent of women affected suffer long-term dysfunction of their fallopian tubes, with resulting infertility or ectopic pregnancy.

PID includes infections of the endometrium, endometritis; the fallopian tubes, salpingitis; the uterine envelope, parametritis; and the inner lining of the pelvis, peritonitis.

In Canada between 1967 and 1977, hospital admissions for PID increased by 50 percent. Increased infertility and ectopic pregnancy occurred during the same period. Ectopic pregnancies expanded from 1 in 246 pregnancies in 1967 to 1 in 147 pregnancies in 1977—a 40 percent increase.

PID is uncommon in women who are not sexually active, and women taking oral contraceptives have a lower incidence of gonococcal PID than women who use no contraception. However, the protective effect of the pill is not well understood. Some researchers avoid using it to prevent PID, since they have not been able to show that it also protects against *Chlamydia*.

What Are the Symptoms of PID?

The symptoms of PID are not particular to this condition. They may include any or all of the following:

1. Deep pain on penetration
2. Nausea and vomiting
3. Cervical or adnexal, i.e., fallopian tube, pain on examination
4. Intermenstrual bleeding or prolonged menstruation
5. Foul smelling discharge
6. Pain on urination

Diagnosis

Diagnostic aids include cultures, smears, and blood work.

Treatment

Most patients with PID can be treated at home with oral antibiotics. Yet, patients are often admitted if they are very ill, pregnant, or if the diagnosis is unclear.

IUDs are usually removed at the first sign of bacterial infection.

Patients are started on antibiotics. If hospitalized, they require intravenous, antimicrobial therapy.

Patients' sexual contacts are treated, and patients are reminded to avoid intercourse until advised differently by their physicians. Failure to adhere to these suggestions will result in reinfection.

About 15 percent of women fail to respond to initial treatment. Twenty percent have recurrences and, as mentioned earlier, 15 percent become infertile as a result of the disease.

Sequelae of PID

Almost all women develop persistent abdominal pain after successful treatment of PID. Laparoscopy usually reveals adhesions in the area of the ovaries. This pain is usually mild and intermittent but occasionally may be severe and disabling.

Infertility

As previously noted, infertility can occur in approximately 15 percent of patients with PID. This is caused by residual scarring of the fallopian tubes, rendering them incapable of successcessfully transfering eggs to the uterus. The risk of such tubal occlusion after one, two, three or more attacks of PID are 12.8 percent, 35.5 percent and 75 percent respectively.

Ectopic Pregnancy

The rising rate of ectopic pregnancy throughout the world is associated with the increased use of IUDs and therefore, the increasing prevalence of PIDs. A woman who has suffered from PID has a six to tenfold greater risk of experiencing an ectopic pregnancy.

An ectopic pregnancy occurs when an egg is fertilized but then is unable to make its way to the uterus for implantation because of dysfunction or scarring of the fallopian tubes. The abnormally placed pregnancy is not viable and must be terminated because it may be a threat to the woman's life.

Pelvic Abscess

This is another consequence of PID, and the abscess must be surgically drained. Occasionally, infection is so extensive that the uterus and the ovaries have to be removed. This is a very uncommon consequence of the disease.

Prevention

PIDs occur as complications of vaginal infections; these, in turn, are caused by certain bacterial organisms. Infection and subsequent disease are best prevented by:

1. Reducing the number of casual sexual encounters
2. Using condoms with spermicidal gels until two people have established a committed relationship and may safely consider another form of contraception, if they wish
3. Giving prompt attention to abnormal vaginal discharge or pelvic pain

Further Reading

Bowie WR. Vaginitis and cervicitis. Med N Am, Infect 2, 1983; 506–510.

Boyd ME. Pelvic inflammatory disease and the general surgeon. Can J Surg 1985; 28:11–13.

Holmes KK, et al. Sexually transmitted disease. New York: McGraw-Hill, 1984; 220–229, 615–632, 763–773.

Lossick JG. Sexually transmitted vaginitis. Urol Clin North Am 1984; 11:141–153.

Muir DG, Belsey MA. Pelvic inflammatory disease and its consequences in the developing world. Am J Obstet Gynecol 1980; 138:913–928.

White FM. Role of prostitution in sexually transmitted disease. Can Med Assoc J 1984; 130:253.

ENTEROPATHOGENS

A number of parasites transmitted from the genital or anal areas to the mouth can ultimately colonize the human bowel. Some organisms are classified as commensals, meaning they pose no danger to the host. Other organisms such as *Giardia lamblia*, resulting in the infection giardiasis, and *Entamoeba histolytica*, resulting in amebiasis, may lead to serious conditions.

Although these diseases may be sexually transmitted, they are usually contracted from infected food handlers or contaminated water supplies. They are most common among homosexuals whose habits include oral-genital and occasionally oral-anal contact. The increased flatulence and diarrhea associated with these diseases have given the condition the name the "Gay Bowel Syndrome."

Giardiasis

The prevalence rate of *Giardia lamblia* in man generally is between 3 and 10 percent; studies of male homosexual communities have found *Giardia lamblia* cysts in 18 percent of those tested. Symptoms are usually mild, consisting of diarrhea that is greasy and buoyant, evictations with a sulfer odor, weight loss and decreased appetite.

Isolation of the organisms may be difficult. Oral medications are often initiated if the presence of *Giardia lamblia* is suspected. Agents used in the treatment of giardiasis include metronidazole (Flagyl) and antabrine (Quinacrine).

Amebiasis

Entamoeba histolytica causes more dramatic symptoms in some of its hosts. Diarrhea may be severe, explosive and bloody. The parasite is usually acquired as a result of foreign travel, but sexual transmission by oral-fecal contamination is well documented and most common in the male homosexual community. Many victims are asymptomatic and so continue unknowingly to spread the disease, amebiasis, to sexual partners. The prevalence in the homosexual community is about 30 percent.

Isolation of *Entamoeba* is achieved by stool sampling, usually three samples, isolation of ova and parasites. As with *Giardia*, the presence of other organisms not usually found in the human digestive tracct, in the absence of *Entamoeba histolytica*, may cause a physician to suspect failure of isolation of the latter, and treatment with metronidazole or other medications may be initiated.

Entamoeba histolytica could also cause infection outside the intestinal tract. The most common complication is liver abscesses. This may be dangerous, and the infection may spread beyond the liver to involve the lining of the lungs, heart or abdomen.

Cryptosporidiosis

Cryptosporidia usually causes a self-limiting infection of the intestinal tract. But in patients with AIDS it may be life threatening; no specific therapy is available for a treatment.

Shigella, *Campylobacter jejuni* and *Strongyloides* are other bowel pathogens, i.e., organisms that may be transmited sexually. They occur infrequently and they are important to consider when oral-anal sex is practiced.

Precautions

When dealing with any bowel pathogens, the sexual contacts of the affected person must be treated as well. Food handlers cannot resume work until repeated cultures are negative. Family members and roommates must also be treated.

Oral-genital and oral-anal contact should be avoided, except within monogamous relationships. Homosexual couples should undergo screening to rule out the presence of these organisms. Patients complaining of diarrhea who have traveled to endemic areas, or who are at risk because of their sexual habits, should have stool sampling for lab culture, as well as examination for ova and parasites.

Further Reading

Guerrant RL, Ravdin JI. Giardia lamblia and Entamoeba histolytica. In: Holmes KK, et al, eds. Sexually transmitted diseases. New York: McGraw-Hill, 1984; 537–553.

Kragstad DJ, et al. Amebiasis. N Engl J Med 1978; 298:262.

Meyers JD, et al. Giardia lamblia infection in homosexual men. Br J Vener Dis 1977; 53:54.

Schmerin MJ, et al. Giardiasis: association with homosexuality. Ann Intern Med 1978; 88:801.

William DC, et al. High rates of enteric protozoal infections in selected homosexual men attending a venereal disease clinic. Sex Transm Dis 1978; 5:155.

GLOSSARY

AIDS: Acquired Immunodeficiency Syndrome

amine: any organic compound containing nitrogen

amyl nitrite: a volatile, inflammable liquid inhalant used in the past as a vasodilator for coronary artery disease; now its derivatives are used for short-lasting "highs."

anaerobic: having the ability to live and grow in the absence of oxygen

anesthesia: loss of sensation in a part or the whole of the body, generally induced by the administration of a drug

androgenic: pertaining to any steroid hormone that promotes male characteristics, namely androsterone and testosterone

aneurysm: a sac-like expansion of a blood-vessel wall

anilingus: sexual activity involving tongue and anus

anorexia nervosa: a condition characterised by extreme aversion to food, usually occurring in young women and resulting in severe weight loss and starvation

antibody: a specific substance produced by the body in response to the presence of an antigen

anticoagulant: a substance that inhibits the action of blood clotting mechanism

antigen: a substance recognized by the body as not being itself, and thereby stimulating cells to produce antibodies

arteriosclerosis: a condition in which the walls of arteries thicken and lose their elasticity; also referred to as "hardening of the arteries"

arthralgia: pain in a joint

arthritis: inflammation of a joint; commonly refers to any disease which involves pain or stiffness of the musculoskeletal system

asymptomatic: showing no symptoms

atherosclerosis: a condition in which fatty substances accumulate abnormally on the inner linings of arteries

autoreproduction: replication; the ability of a gene or virus to synthesize another molecule like itself from smaller molecules within the cell

balanitis:	inflammation of the glans penis or "head" of the penis, producing a red and occasionally coated surface
bartholinitis:	inflammation of the Bartholin glands, two small glands one on each side of the vaginal opening, secreting mucus
basal body temperature:	base level temperature for any given person considered as their normal body temperature upon awakening, before physical activity, and when free of disease
benign:	not malignant; favoring recovery
bulbourethral:	pertaining to the bulb of the urethra
Campylobacter:	a genus of bacteria of the family *Spirillaceae*, made up of gram negative, non- spore forming, motile, spirally curved rods, which are microaerophilic to anaerobic
Candida albicans:	yeast-like fungi that are commonly part of the normal flora of the mouth, skin, intestinal tract, vagina, but that can cause a variety of infections
cardiovascular disease:	any disease pertaining to the heart and its tributaries (arteries)
cervicitis:	inflammation of the mucous membrane of the cervix
cervix:	the narrow, inferior end of the uterus that leads into the vagina
chancre:	the primary lesion of syphilis occurring at the site of entry of the infection, usually painless with raised edges and at times, ulcerated
chemotherapy:	the treatment of illness by drugs; esp. for cancer
Chlamydia:	a primitive form of bacteria which acts as an obligate intracellular parasite to cause many diseases in vertebrate animals
chloasma:	hyperpigmentation in certain limited areas of the skin, esp. during pregnancy; also called the "mask of pregnancy"
chorion:	the embryonic membrane that forms the outermost covering around a developing fetus and contributes to the formation of the placenta
chorionic gonadotropin:	a hormone secreted by the placenta during gestation
chromosome:	a structure in the cell nucleus which contains the genes necessary for heredity
cirrhosis:	a progressive degenerate disease of the liver, frequently resulting in jaundice, liver failure, coma, and death
clitoris:	a small, erectile organ located in the anterior portion of the female vulva, corresponding to the penis in the male, and aiding in the female orgasm
CNS:	the Central Nervous System, consisting of the brain and spinal cord

collagen: a protein occurring in the white fibres of connective tissue, cartilage, and in the matrix of bone

colposcopy: examination of the vagina and cervix by means of a magnifying lens, used for the early detection of malignant changes

commensalism: a relationship in which one member benefits and the other is uneffected in any way

condyloma: an elevated wart-like lesion of the skin or mucosa, found in the areas of the mouth, penis, vulva, vagina, anus, or rectum

congenital: any condition that exists at the time of birth

conjunctivitis: inflammation of the membrane which lines the eyelids and covers the eyeball

corpus cavernosum: either of the two columns of erectile tissue forming the body of the penis or clitoris

corpus luteum: a yellow, glandular mass in the ovary formed by an ovarian follicle that has matured and discharged its ovum

corpus spongiosum: a column of erectile tissue forming the urethral surface of the penis in the urethra is found

Cowper's glands: also the bulbourethral glands

cremaster muscle: the muscle that elevates the testis

cryotherapy: the use of cold by liquid nitrogen at near absolute zero, in the treatment of disease

Cryptococcus: a genus of yeast-like fungi

crystal violet: a basic aniline dye used to inactivate nucleic acids; thought to be useful in the treatment of fungal skin infections and vaginal infections caused by yeasts and gram negative bacteria

cutaneous anergy: a diminished sensitivity of the skin to specific antigens

cystitis: inflammation of the urinary bladder

cytology: the anatomy, physiology, pathology, and chemistry of the cell

cytomegalovirus: a group of herpes viruses infecting man and animals; they are all species specific

cytotoxic: destructive to cells

desensitization: the reduction of allergic sensitivity or reactions to the specific antigen

desquamate: to shed, peel, or scale off, as in the shedding of the epidermis in scales or sheets

disseminated gonococcal infection: gonorrhea infection that has spread from its origin (area of contact) throughout the body

douche: a stream of water or air directed against a part of a body or into a cavity; eg. vaginal douche

dysfunctional: having difficult or abnormal function; i.e. abnormal, out of the ordinary vaginal bleeding

dysmenorrhea: difficult or painful menstruation

ectoparasite: a parasite that lives on the surface of the body

ectopic pregnancy: pregnancy in which the fertilized ovum becomes implanted outside the uterus instead of in the walls of the uterus; also referred to as "extrauterine pregnancy"

electrocautery: cauterization of tissue by means of an electrode

encephalitis: inflammation of the brain

endocarditis: inflammation of the endocardium, the innermost lining of the heart

endometritis: inflammation of the endometrium, the innermost lining of the uterus

endoparasite: a parasite which lives within the body of its host

enteric: relating to the intestine

epidemiology: the science of epidemics and epidemic diseases

epilepsy: a chronic disorder characterized by paroxysmal attacks of brain dysfunction, usually associated with some alteration of consciousness

erythromycin: a broad spectrum antibiotic produced by a strain of *Streptomyces erythreus*

estrogen: the female sex hormones, formed in the ovary, adrenal cortex, testis, and fetoplacental unit; responsible for the secondary sex characteristics and for preparation of the uterus for pregnancy

etiology: the study of the causes of disease

exudate: a fluid of protein and cellular debris which has escaped from blood vessels and has been deposited in tissues or tissue surfaces, usually as a result of inflammation

FDA: Food and Drug Administration; an agency of the Department of Health, Education, and Welfare which enforces the Federal Food, Drug, and Cosmetic Act

febrile: pertaining to fever

fibrocystic: characterized by an overgrowth of fibrous tissue and the development of cystic spaces, esp. in a gland

fibroid: having a fibrous structure resembling a fibroid (tumor composed mainly of fibrous or fully developed connective tissue

follicle: a sac or pouch-like depression or cavity

frenulum: a small fold of integument or mucous membrane that limits the movement of an organ or part; f. of clitoris; f. of prepuce of penis

FSH: follicle stimulating hormone; one of the gonadotropic hormones of the anterior lobe of the pituitary gland that stimulates growth and maturation of graafian follicles in the ovary and stimulates spermatogenesis in the testis

fulminant: occurring suddenly and with great intensity

functional: pertaining to or fulfilling a function; affecting the function but not the structure

gammaglobulin: a class of plasma proteins composed almost entirely of immunoglobulins, the proteins that function as antibodies

gastroenteritis: inflammation of the lining of the stomach and intestine

gastrointestinal: pertaining to the stomach and intestine

Giardia lamblia: a species of flagellate protozoa parasitic in the intestines of man

giardiasis: infection with *Giardia lamblia*

glomerulonephritis: a variety of kidney disease

gonadotropic: stimulating the gonads; referring to the hormones of the anterior pituitary gland which influence the gonads

gonorrhea: a highly contagious bacterial infection by the organism *Neisseria gonorrhoeae*, usually of the female or male genital tracts, but as well of the oral or anal cavities

Guillain-Barré syndrome: a relatively rare disease affecting the peripheral nervous system, esp. in the spinal nerves (resulting in temporary "paralysis")

hemophiliac: a person inflicted with hemophilia, a condition characterized by impaired coagulability of the blood and a strong tendency to bleed

hepatitis: inflammation of the liver

herpes: any inflammatory skin disease caused by a herpesvirus and characterized by the forma tion of small vesicles in clusters

HTLV-III: Human T-lymphotropic virus

hymen: the membranous fold partly or completely closing the vaginal orifice

hypertension: persistently high blood pressure; chronically exceeding 140/90 mm Hg.

hypothalamus: the portion of the diencephalon lying beneath the thalamus at the base of the cerebrum

idoxuridine: a pyrimidine analogue that prevents replication of DNA viruses; used topically in herpes simplex keratitis

immunity: the condition of being immune; nonsusceptibility to the pathogenic effects of foreign microorganisms or to the toxic effects of antigenic substances

immunofluoresence: the use of fluorescein-labeled antibodies to identify specific bacterial, viral, or other antigenic material specific for the labeled antibody

immunosuppression: inhibition of the formation of antibodies to antigens that may be present; used in transplantation procedures to prevent rejection of the transplanted organ or tissue

infibulation: stitching together the lips of the vulva or of the prepuce in order to prevent copulation

inguinal canal: the oblique passage in the lower anterior abdominal wall, through which passes the round ligament of the uterus in the female, and the spermatic cord in the male

insufflate: to blow powder, vapor, or gas into a body cavity

interferon: a natural glycoprotein released by cells invaded by viruses; it is not itself an antiviral agent, but rather acts as a stimulant to non-infected cells, causing them to synthesize another protein with antiviral characteristics

interstitial: pertaining to or situated between parts or in the interspaces of tissues

introitus: the entrance into a canal or hollow organ, as the vagina

jaundice: yellowness of the skin, sclerae, mucous membranes, and excretions due to excessive deposition of bile pigments

Kaposi's sarcoma: a multifocal, metastasizing, malignant cancer involving mainly the skin

labia majora: elongated folds in the female, one on either side of the opening to the vagina lateral to the labia minora

labia minora: the small folds of skin on either side of the labia majora and the opening of the vagina

laparoscopy: examination of the peritoneal cavity by means of a laparoscope through a small incision in the area of the umbilicus

latency: a state of being dormant or concealed

LAV: lymphadenopathy associated virus

LH: luteinizing hormone; a gonadotropic hormone of the anterior pituitary gland acting with FSH to cause ovulation of mature follicles and estrogen secretion; is also concerned with the formation of the corpus luteum; in males, LH stimulates development of the interstitial cells of the testes and testosterone secretion

lymphadenopathy syndrome: disease of the lymph nodes, causing generalized enlargement of lymph nodes throughout the body

malignant hyperthermia: a syndrome affecting patients undergoing general anesthesia marked by a rapid rise in body temperature, signs of increased muscle metabolism, and often

	rigidity; the sensitivity is inherited as an autosomal dominant trait
meiosis:	the process of cell division by which reproductive cells (gametes) are formed
menarche:	the beginning of the menstrual cycle; first menstruation
meningitis:	inflammation of the meninges of the brain and spinal cord
metronidazole:	an orally effective trichomonicide used in the treatment of infections caused by *Trichomonas vaginalis*
molluscum contagiosum:	an infectious disease of the skin caused by a virus characterized by the appearance of small, papular epithelial lesions which contain "molluscum bodies"
mons pubis:	the prominence caused by a pad of fat over the symphysis pubis in the female
morbidity:	the condition of being diseased
Mycobacterium:	a genus of gram-negative bacteria characterized by acid-fast staining
Mycostatin:	the trademark for a preparation of nystatin, an antifungal agent
myocardial infarction:	necrosis of the cells of an area of the heart muscle (myocardium) occurring as a result of oxygen deprivation, which in turn is caused by obstruction to the blood supply; commonly referred to as "heart attack"
necrosis:	cell death
Neisseria gonorrhoeae:	the etiologic agent of gonorrhea
neoplasia:	the formation of a neoplasm (tumor); any new and abnormal growth
neuralgia:	pain in a nerve or along the course of one or more nerves
neurosyphilis:	syphilis affecting the nervous system
obligate:	not facultative; necessary; compulsory; characterized by the ability to survive only in a particular environment or to assume only a particular role
ophthalmia neonatorium:	any hyperacute purulent conjunctivitis, e.g., gonorrheal ophthalmia
opportunistic:	pertaining to a microorganism which does not ordinarily cause disease but which becomes pathogenic under certain circumstances
oral candidiasis:	infection, by fungi of the genus *Candida*, of the oral mucosa
otitis media:	inflammation of inner ear, occurring most often in infants and young children
papillomavirus:	causative virus of condylomata lata or venereal warts

Papanicolaou test:	a simple, painless test used most commonly to detect cancer of uterus. and cervix (PAP test)
pathogenic:	causing disease
pediculosis pubis:	infestation with lice of the species *Phthirus pubis*, the crab louse, of the pubic hairs, and occasionally, of the eyelashes, eyebrows, axillae hairs
perineum:	the area between the thighs extending from the coccyx to the pubis and lying below the pelvic diaphragm
peripheral neuropathy:	referring to functional disturbances and pathologic changes in the peripheral nervous system
peritonitis:	inflammation of the perineum
periumbilical:	around the umbilicus
pessary:	an instrument placed in the vagina to support the uterus or rectum or as a contraceptive device
pituitary gland:	an endocrine gland located at the base of the brain; commonly referred to as the "master gland"
placebo:	an indifferent substance, in the form of medicine, given for its suggestive effect
placenta:	the organ of interchange between the fetus and the mother
pleurisy:	inflammation of the pleura (lining of the lungs)
pneumonitis:	inflammation of the lung tissue
podophyllum:	the dried root and rhizome of Podophyllum peltatum, used as a topical caustic in the treatment of certain papillomas (venereal warts)
post-pill amenorrhea:	absence of menses
proctitis:	inflammation of the mucous membrane of the rectum
proctoscopy:	examination of the rectum with a proctoscope
prodrome:	a premonitory symptom; one indicating the onset of a disease
progesterone:	a steroid hormone that is the main hormone of pregnancy; it also plays a role in the menstrual cycle
prophylactic:	tending to ward off disease; to prevent
prostaglandin:	a class of physiologically active substances present in many tissues; their effects include mainly uterine stimulation
prostate gland:	a gland in the male which surrounds the neck of the bladder and the urethra
protozoan:	pertaining to unicellular, eucaryotic organisms
quinine:	a white, flaky, odorless bitter powder used as an antimalarial agent
retrovirus:	a large group of RNA viruses that includes the leukoviruses and lentiviruses

salpingitis:	inflammation of the uterine tube (fallopian tube)
Sarcoptes scabiei:	the "itch" mite; the cause of scabies in man
seminiferous tubules:	the tubules of the testes which produce and carry semen
sensitivity:	the state of being able to respond to a stimulus
sequelae:	morbid conditions following or occurring as a consequence of another illness
seropositive:	showing positive results on serologic examination
Shigella:	a genus of bacteria that cause dysentery
smegma:	secretion of the sebaceous glands; s. clitoris; s. preputii
specificity:	the state of having a fixed relation to a single cause; for example, of an antibody to its antigen
spermatogenesis:	the process of formation and development of the spermatozoan
spermatogonium:	the primitive sperm "mother" cell which divides to form the spermatocyte
STD:	sexually transmitted disease
spermicide:	an agent destructive to spermatazoa
Strongyloides:	a genus of nematode parasites often found in the small intestine of herbivorous animals
symbiosis:	a relationship between two organisms in which both benefit from the coexistence
syphilis:	an acute, chronic, and infectious disease caused by *Treponema pallidum*, and usually transmitted by sexual contact
teratogenic:	causing abnormal development in the developing embryo
tetracycline:	a broad spectrum antibiotic
thromboembolism:	an embolism from a thrombus dislodged from a vein
thrombophlebitis:	inflammation of a vein associated with thrombus formation
thrombosis:	formation or development of a clot in a blood vessel, or in a heart cavity
thrush:	an infection of the oral mucosa by a fungus, characterized by a red, inflamed surface with white patches, and accompanied by pain and fever
T-lymphocyte:	a type of white cell required for the regulation of the immune system and defence of the body against foreign tumors and virus infected cells; also referred to as a "T-cell"
toxemia:	the condition occurring as a result of the spread of bacterial toxins by the bloodstream
toxoplasmosis:	a disease due to *Toxoplasma gondi*
trachoma:	a chronic, contagious viral inflammation of the conjunctiva, caused by *Chlamydia trachomatis*
transplacental:	crossing the placenta

Treponema pallidum: a genus of spirochetes which is parasitic for man and other animals; the etiologic agent of syphilis

trichloroacetic acid: an extremely caustic acid used in medicine as a topical caustic for lesions

trichomoniasis: an STD caused by *Trichomonas vaginalis*; in females, infections may be either asymptomatic or symptomatic, accompanied by itching and burning; males can be asymptomatic carriers

tubal ligation: a term used for various operative procedures that involve the cutting, cauterization, or ligation of the fallopian tubes to achieve permanent sterilization in women

tuberculosis: a chronic, infectious disease which commonly affects the lungs

urethra: the canal leading from the bladder which externally discharges the urine

vaginal rugae: many transverse ridges or folds found in the mucous membrane of the vagina

vaginitis: inflammation of the vagina

varicose veins: swollen and distended veins found commonly in the subcutaneous tissues of the leg often resulting from a sluggish flow of blood or from weakened venous walls

vasa deferentia: the excretory ducts of the testes which joins the excretory duct of the seminal vesicle, forming the ejaculatory duct

vasectomy: surgical interruption of the vas deferens to cause sterility in men

vasa efferentia: vessels which direct fluid away from an area

venereal warts: a lay term used for *Condylomata accuminata*, an infection by papillomaviruses

vulva: the external genital organs of the female

INDEX

The letter f following a page number indicates a figure; the letter t following a page number indicates a table.